The
Scandinavian
Diet

Dr Sofie Hexeberg

The Scandinavian Diet

**Getting Healthy
with Low Carb**

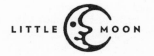

LITTLE MOON

Published by Little Moon Publishing Ltd.,
Third Floor, Premier House
12–13 Hatton Garden
London EC1N 8AN
UNITED KINGDOM
www.littlemoonpublishing.com

ISBN 978-1-90801802-1

Text copyright Cappelen Damm © 2011
First English edition 2012
Translated from Norwegian by Charles Ek
Based upon the Norwegian edition "Frisk med lavkarbo"
Designed in Norway
Printed by Nørhaven in Denmark
Cover design by Mette Gundersen, Norway

Thank you

It was my husband, Erik, who encouraged me to write this book. He is himself a physician and has listened patiently and with great wonder and enthusiasm when I talk about the fantastic results my patients have achieved when they changed to a low carbohydrate diet. He supported me during the writing process and pointed out how important it is that this message reaches more people.

After reading a great deal about the low carbohydrate diet, I started to work at Dr. Fedon A. Lindberg's clinic. Fedon shared his knowledge and experience with me, and his enthusiasm for the significance of diet for health and well-being has been a great inspiration. Fedon invited me to be part of forming The Society for Dietary Reform to Alleviate Diabetes and Other Diseases (Foreningen kostreform ved overvekt og sukkersykdommer) which is how I became acquainted with Dag Viljen Poleszynski, who for years has worked to promote the Stone Age diet. Dag is like a living library in this field, and he has given me a great deal of new insight and stimulated me to study the literature in this area. He has provided me with professional support during this writing process, for which I am very grateful.

A big thank you also to my editor Lise Galaasen at Cappelen Damm. She was extremely positive when I presented my idea of writing this book. She encouraged me and has been my midwife – I couldn't have managed without her.

And I especially want to thank all of my patients, from whom I have learned so much and who have stimulated me to seek more knowledge about their diseases and health problems. If I had not received feedback from the patients and seen the effects of a low carbohydrate diet in practice, I would not have believed it to be possible. A special thank you to the patients who allowed me to use their stories in this book.

Dr Sofie Hexeberg
www.drhexeberg.no

Contents

Introduction

This book is based on patients I have treated with a low carb diet and is an expression of my understanding of how food works in our bodies. I have acquired this understanding over many years, and it is based on my own experiences with patients and the research and experience of a number of other physicians. I have come to realize that it is too many carbohydrates, not too much fat, that is the main cause of many of our lifestyle diseases. A low carb diet is the way to go for the great majority who struggle with insulin resistance and being overweight .

All the patients have given their consent to being part of the book, and all of them have been given a new name. The common features in most of the case histories are of patients being overweight and having high insulin levels, which leads to several biochemical and hormonal problems. This again results in many diseases and health problems. The case histories that I present are typical of what I meet in my practice. Some may wonder why I don't document this through research. My reply is that this type of study requires a lot of money that is hard to get. Besidies, it requires a great deal of time, and I have chosen to use my time directly on the patients who need my knowledge. They don't have time to wait for more studies; they need help now.

Imagine that you were a doctor before WWII. Pneumonia was a common disease, but you didn't have medicines that would cure the disease, and many died. Then you got access to penicillin and started treating patients with new medicine. To your great joy, the first patient regained their health, the second and the third as well. When you had cured 50 patients with penicillin, you were quite convinced that this medicine worked. Surely you wouldn't have needed to read ten double blind studies that said penicillin makes people with pneumonia healthy?

I have done research previously and have a Ph.D. I have read thousands of articles, many of which show that a low carb diet is beneficial for people with obesity and other diseases. The objection is that there are no long-term studies. The longest study yet ran for two years, and it shows that those whose diet contained a lot of fat and few carbohydrates had better results regarding weight reduction and fats in the blood than those who ate low calorie, low fat food.

Before the agricultural revolution, our ancestors lived for about two million years on a diet composed of few carbohydrates. In other words, millions of people have had experience eating this way right up to our time. In recent years, there are many examples of people who have lived on a low carb diet for even decades, with very good results. Among the many examples, we find anthropologist Vilhjalmur Stefansson, doctors Wolfgang Lutz, Jan Kwasniewski, Robert Atkins and Robert K. Su, and nutrition experts Barry Groves, Dag Viljen Poleszynski, Iver Mysterud and Jonny Laupsa-Borge.

Besides, the burden of proof actually lies on the authorities who tell us that we must eat the high carb, low fat food, which is leading to more people becoming overweight and getting diabetes. Humans have evolved over several million years, and for most of that time they ate neither bread, rice, pasta, tortillas, ready-made food nor sweets. They ate what they found in nature, which was mainly meat, fish, shellfish, eggs, nuts, seeds, insects, vegetables, fruit and berries. That is the food we were made to eat. Only birds can eat raw grain – we're not designed for that.

If you live according to the advice of public health or worse, I recommend that you reduce your consumption of carbohydrates. If you have insulin resistance, obesity and type 2 diabetes, it is absolutely vital. Some people like fat and prefer to eat a diet in which fat makes up approximately 80 percent of their energy intake. Experience has shown that this is completely justifiable health-wise. However, some people don't do well with that much fat and prefer getting about 50 percent of their energy in the form of fat with somewhat more protein and carbohydrates. When we reduce our consumption of carbohydrates, our consumption of fat must necessarily increase, because there are limits to how much protein we can manage to eat. When we eat too much protein, the surplus is, in fact, converted to sugar, which is not good either.

On September 2, 2009, Norwegian nutrition authorities stated on a television news programme that a low carb diet may be an alternative treatment for overweight and obesity. They based their statement on the existing studies of low-carb diets. It came as a great surprise and is a milestone in official Norwegian dietary recommendations. It is beneficial not only in order to battle overweight, but for a range of other conditions that you will read about in this book.

Experience

My own professional development and dietary history

When I was 16 years old, I started to get interested in the food we eat. My motivation at that time was that, like all girls of that age, I had put on a little more fat on my body. Not that I was fat, but I always thought I should to be 2 to 3 kilograms (4 to 6 pounds) lighter. I wasn't the only one, of course – almost all girls of my age dieted periodically. It was popular to be thin, and we didn't want to have too many curves. It was all about fasting, protein diets, tomato diets and other starvation diets. But the desire for food always increased after these diets, and the weight that had disappeared came right back.

The summer I was 19, I put on 10 kilograms (1 stone 8). Which wasn't so strange, because I ate lots of bread, cakes, ice cream and chocolate. I didn't feel well, neither physically or psychologically. None of my clothes fit, I felt less attractive and I stayed home most of the time. In the course of the next six months, however, I lost the extra weight again, and life became easier.

During my first pregnancy, I put on 20 kilograms (3 stone 2), which is far too much. The reason again was, of course, a large consumption of bread and sweets. After the delivery, I was left with 15 kilograms (2 stone 5) of extra fat. With the help of willpower, I got rid of the weight and vowed to never let it happen again. During the following pregnancies, I put on only 8 to 10 kilograms (17–22 pounds). As I read more and more about the impact of diet on health, I became more and more interested.

When my medical studies were completed, I was awarded funds for a research project. I studied the effects of fat, fibre and cholesterol in food; on fats in the blood and the heart; and their effects on the heart's function. The experiments were carried out on rats and rabbits, but research results from animals cannot be applied directly to humans. During this period, however, I read about the dangers of fat and cholesterol. I did this for five years until I presented my doctoral thesis for the Doctor Medicinæ degree (Dr. Med.). During this period I became a vegetarian, because it seemed sensible after everything I had read about how dangerous fat was and how healthy fibre was. A vegetarian diet suited me well because I was very fond of bread, and as a child I always preferred potatoes with gravy over meat and fish. I made my own bread from whole wheat flour, because that was so healthy. In addition to this, my diet consisted of potatoes, rice, pasta, lots of vegetables and fruit and low fat dairy products. For 15 years I seldom ate eggs and never meat, fowl, fish or shellfish. I tried various vegetarian diets because I was preoccupied with finding the optimal way to eat. I tried, for example, eaiting only fruit, which I only managed for a few week because I was always hungry and had an enormous craving for sugar because of my fluctuating blood sugar. During another period, I ate only raw food consisting mainly of vegetables, fruit, berries, nuts and vegetable juices. That wasn't a simple diet either and had to be discarded.

While doing my doctoral studies, I worked in the pathology department of a Norwegian hospital, where, among other things, I conducted autopsies. When I saw all of the fat that some people had in their arteries, I became even more convinced that a low fat diet was the only way to avoid cardiovascular disease. I worked in a diabetes department as well, and saw how patients with type 1 and type 2 diabetes struggled to control their blood sugar. I did as I had been taught – explained that they needed to eat low fat foods because they had an increased risk of getting cardiovascular disease. Medications were prescribed in rapid succession. I worked a couple of years in a company health service, where I put my heart and soul into preventative work, especially regarding food. Oily fish was OK; otherwise, everything was to be low fat, and the bread was to be coarse. For a period I also worked at the Norwegian Medicines Agency, where I evaluated many pharmaceuticals and informed doctors about their use. When you investigate the numbers in such studies carefully, you are surprised by how little effect many such medications have. For each patient that experiences a positive effect, there are often many patients for whom the medicines have no effect, while some only get the side effects.

Then Fedon Lindberg (a Norwegian physician who advocates a low carb diet) arrived on the scene and turned everything on its head. I read many books and articles by doctors and other therapists who told of the unbelievable effects their patients achieved when they reduced their consumption of carbohydrates and ate more fat. All this really got me thinking. I recognised finally that I had been completely wrong. Humans have never been vegetarians: the optimal diet is the hunter-gatherer diet that humans have lived on for several million years.

So it was time to try a new diet, and I got started a winter holiday in the mountains. I cut out virtually all carbohydrates, so that my diet consisted of meat, fish, eggs, cheese and a few vegetables that grow above the ground. After a couple of days, my stockpiled store of sugar was emptied, and I could barely stand on my feet. I was unbelievably weak, had a headache and cramps in my feet and was afraid I wouldn't live to the next day. So I had a piece of fruit, and that helped a little. It was impossible to go skiing with the children, so I discontinued the diet. I tried again later, and the same thing happened. My body had, of course, lived on sugar for 15 years and forgotten how to metabolise fat.

I decided to proceed a little more gradually. Little by little, I reduced the number of carbohydrates I ingested, until I ate approximately 50 grams per day. I got these carbohydrates mostly from vegetables, berries, nuts and dairy products without added sugar. I felt fine. Many of the problems I used to have, such as a bloated stomach, hyperacidity, wolfish hunger and sweet cravings, disappeared. Moreover, I became more at peace with myself and my disposition became more stable. My hairdresser wondered what I had been doing lately. I didn't understand what she meant, and she said that thousands of new hairs were growing in my scalp. This happened shortly after I had begun the new diet, and I interpreted it as my body finally having the strength and nutrients to give me a little fuller hair.

The years have brought me much knowledge and experience, and now I place more emphasis on my own experiences and reflections when faced with the jungle of existing "official information". I have quite simply begun to rely more on myself and no longer take everything as gospel truth, regardless of whether it comes from on high in the scientific world. Interpretations of new data in scientific circles are made in light of the prevailing thoughts and while research-ers often cling to this, outsiders can more readily see that the prevailing understanding must be changed. A professor I had at university said the following before a lecture: "Half of what I am teaching you now is wrong – it's just too bad that I don't know which half." If everyone were this honest with regard to knowledge, a lot of things would look diffe-rent.

Patient experience

Gradually I had acquired a lot of theoretical knowledge about the low carb diet and had experienced the positive effects on my own body. The time was now ripe to treat patients with this diet to see if all of this was right. And it was! Everything I had read about and experienced myself – and more – worked on the patients I treated. I was quite simply shocked that the diet could have such potent effects, and I decided that this would be my working platform the rest of my life.

Many patients look confused when I say that they can cook with butter, cream and sour cream. It goes against everything they have previously learned from authorities and weight-loss experts. They never eat butter, they use skimmed milk and low fat cheese, they cut away all visible fat from their meat, eat chicken fillets frequently and use a lot of low calorie foods. But even though they've eaten low fat food, they've become overweight. I ask them to forget everything they have learned about diet for a couple of months and follow my advice. This, of course, is why they have come to me in the first place.

Bread is the most difficult food to avoid. Without bread,

people ask, what am I to eat for breakfast, lunch and supper? I suggest eating an omelette with fresh vegetables for breakfast. Many think that's fine, but after a month they're tired of omelettes; they need variety. They've been eating a slice of bread with cheese and one with jam for 40 years, but that they haven't become tired of. Though it may seen strange, it demonstrates how we like our routines and have difficulty in changing our habits. For those who need variety, I give them for example a recipe for low carb protein bread, pancakes or tips on crisp bread that has reduced carbohydrates. Things usually go well after that. And anyway, it's possible to continue having omelettes for breakfast – eventually, this will become a new habit you won't want to break.

So what about lunch? What do we have for lunch instead of a sandwich? I suggest a salad with chicken or tuna instead. Those who have a nice cafeteria at work think this is splendid. Others have to make the salad themselves and say they don't have time for that. I ask how many hours they watch TV each day. Then most people realise that they have time after all. For all of us, it's a matter of prioritising how to use our time. Moreover, it doesn't take very many minutes to make lunch if we always make plenty of food for dinner. Then it's just a matter of putting the leftovers in a container in the refrigerator, and tomorrow's lunch is ready.

Most people think it's relatively easy to eat a dinner without potatoes, rice or pasta. They just use more vegetables instead. Some think they have to have some pulses or peas now and then, and that's fine in moderation, since pulses give only a low increase of blood sugar. Many people have sweet cravings and need to put something nice in their mouths in the evening. For these people, I suggest that they instead eat a small meal. Some overweight people need to eat even when they aren't hungry, but of course that won't lead to any great weight loss. If you want to eat when you're not hungry, it should absolutely be something that is low in carbohydrates and low in calories, like vegetables, possibly with a little dip.

Everyone needs to have a good time on the weekends, and the weekend lasts almost half the week – from Friday to Monday. It's actually odd that we need so much satisfaction all at once.

We enjoy ourselves watching a film, but need chocolate or potato crisps at the same time. Isn't it better to enjoy the film and then enjoy something good to eat afterwards? We gain more benefit from both things by doing each on its own. We can unconsciously gobble masses of food while watching TV. You can make sugar-free cakes and desserts and eat bacon crisps instead of potato crisps. Chocolate with 70 or 86 percent cocoa covers the need for sweets and chocolate for many people. In moderate quantities, it's actually healthy because of the high content of anti-oxidants.

I explain to all of my patients the physiological basis for their symptoms. To me it is very important that we all know a little about how the body functions and why it reacts as it does in various situations. I take blood samples from all my patients who need monitoring. Then I review them carefully and explain their significance.

When you visit your general practitioner, a specialist or are in hospital, I recommend you ask questions so that you understand what the various examinations mean. Ask also what you yourself can do to improve your condition. Check out the Internet, read books and discuss with friends and colleagues. That way you will acquire more knowledge and be in a better position to take care of your own body.

Patient case histories

The whole idea behind this book is the patient case histories. When I decided to write the book, I was of course completely dependent on my patients allowing me to tell their stories. These are patients I treated from 2006–2009, and several of them I have not had contact with since 2006. There were 35 different names on the list I had made for myself in the course of these years. I chose these patients because collectively they demonstrate the breadth of ailments a low carbohydrate diet can cure. Most patients came to me primarily to lose weight, but on a carbohydrate-restricted diet many different diseases were also cured or significantly easier to live with.

For various reasons, I was a little reluctant to call people. I wondered whether they remembered me, whether they thought I was being pushy, and whether they had gone back to their previous diet and had seen their health decline. These concerns were fortunately unfounded, for everyone was positive towards the book and wanted to share their story with others in the hope that they too could achieve a better life with the right food. They thought it was exciting to read their own history, and they were reminded of how poor their health had been before they changed their diet.

Thirty-three of the 35 patients I called had maintained the low carbohydrate diet, and were well. Two had gone back to their old diet and got back all the health problems they had before. These two became motivated to return to a low carbohydrate diet after our talk.

The patient case histories contain some blood sample results and medical terms that will be explained the first time they are used. Difficult words and expressions will also be explained in an overview on pages 277–293. After most of the patient case histories, you will find a table with blood sample results. All the blood samples have been taken after an overnight fast. Along with the blood sample results, I provide reference values at the laboratory in question, with the exception of C-peptide and triglycerides, which I think have been set too high in relation to what is desirable (see pages 280–281). Many of the reference ranges are probably far from optimal, but I haven't gone into that in more detail, since we don't know what 'optimal' is. Key concepts in this book are C-peptide and insulin resistance, which are explained on pages 280 and 291.

For the chapters on various diseases, I've written a section on traditional treatment. By this, I mean the treatment that is customarily offered by health officials. The histories in this book show that these patients achieved better results by eating low carb food than they achieved with traditional treatment. Many could discontinue different medicines as a result of their dietary changes.

For most diagnoses, I have many histories similar to those you will read in the book. But I cannot, of course, guarantee that everyone will achieve the same results. How long one has had the disease and the combination of different diseases probably enters into it. Moreover, we are all different, and some of you will need more specific dietary advice and/or diet supplements. However, I will recommend that you try this diet to see how it affects your body. For people with chronic diseases, I recommend monitoring by a physician when making radical dietary changes.

What is it we eat?

What did we eat before?

Grain was introduced to Scandinavia approximately 6000 years ago, but more than 2000 years passed before grain cultivation became particularly widespread. We started to grow potatoes after the middle of the 1700's. Before people ate grain and potatoes, they lived exclusively from hunting, fishing and gathering and were therefore at the mercy of whatever nature offered.

All hunters and gatherers needed to procure more energy than the energy they used to get the food. They had to prioritise what they would catch or gather in relation to how much energy they got for the effort. Hence they preferred large animals to small ones, animal-based food rather than vegetable-based food, and fatty rather than lean food. Since they had to cover their need for vitamins and minerals via the food, they ate almost every part of the animals they caught – unlike us, who mainly eat the muscles. You're wondering perhaps how healthy these people were. Many researchers, missionaries and explorers have studied peoples with lifestyles that haven't been affected by Western culture. Independently of each other, they have pointed out that these people did not suffer from diseases such as cancer, heart attack, diabetes, obesity, tooth decay, eczema and psoriasis. Such diseases emerged after people with a natural lifestyle changed their diet.

People with a natural lifestyle who survived infant mortality, infections, injuries, and who were not eaten by wild animals, lived until they were 90–100 years old. An average life expectancy was, however, lower than today because of the dangerous environment in which they lived. In the same way, wild animals live much longer in zoos than in the wild – they are genetically identical, but protected from danger.

What are we eating now?

The diet of the average person in the Western world today is very different from the Stone Age diet. It contains sugar and starch and consists of a lot of bread, cereal, crisp bread, potatoes, rice, pasta and pizza. Then there is fast food, cakes, rolls, potato crisps, chocolate – not to mention all the sugar we consume via soft drinks, fruit drinks and fresh juice. Furthermore, the quality of the food has worsened considerably over the last century. International experts in agriculture have estimated that the mineral content in North American topsoil has been reduced by 85 percent in 70 years. In Europe, the reduction has been around 72 percent. The trend is the same when it comes to vitamins. This has led to, for example, apples having lost on average 80 percent of their vitamin C content, and the nutritional content of our plant foods is estimated overall to have been halved in the course of two generations.

Below you will find an overview of what our food is composed of. The largest content of the food we eat is called macronutrients and consists of carbohydrates, proteins and fat.

What are carbohydrates?

Carbohydrates is a collective term for sugar, starch, glycogen and fibre, where sugar, starch and glycogen provide energy, while fibre does not. What we call sugar is either a simple or double sugars that are found in our food in their natural form. Starch is the plant world's storage form for sugar and consists of chains that have been put together from the simple sugar-glucose. Animals and humans store sugar in the liver and in muscles in the form of glycogen. Just like starch, glycogen consists of chains put together from glucose. The quantity of glycogen in the liver and muscles is, however, very small, because the most important way for mammals to store energy is fat.

Starch is found in large quantities in grain products, potatoes and other root vegetables. When starch is broken down in the intestine, glucose enters the blood. This happens quickly and causes a substantial elevation of blood sugar levels. Foods that contain a lot of starch should therefore be eaten in limited quantities.

Disaccharides (double sugars) must be broken down by special enzymes in the intestine before the glucose can be absorbed into the blood. All galactose and most fructose is transformed into glucose in the liver. Consequently, you only get 50 percent glucose from common white sugar and lactose through break down in the intestine, whereas malt extract gives 100 percent glucose. That's why you get greatly elevated blood sugar levels after drinking beer, which contains a great deal of maltose. You also get glucose from starch, because starch consists only of glucose molecules. Starch decomposes partially into glucose in the mouth, while the rest is decomposed in the gastrointestinal system.

Type of carbohydrate	Carbohydrate consists of
Simple sugars/Monosaccharides	
Glucose (grape sugar)	Glucose
Fructose (fruit sugar)	Fructose
Galactose	Galactose
Disaccharides	
Sucrose (common white sugar)	Glucose + fructose
Lactose (milk sugar)	Glucose + galactose
Maltose (malt extract)	Glucose + glucose
Polysaccharides	
Starch (pectin, amylopectin)	Glucose-glucose-glucose …
Glycogen	Glucose-glucose-glucose …

The consequence of digestion in the mouth is felt when you chew long enough on a slice of bread; it begins to taste sweet. The point is that the body gets glucose faster from starch than from common white sugar when these carbohydrates are consumed in the same quantity. Consequently, you get higher blood sugar from eating white bread than from eating sugar!

What does the body use carbohydrates for, and what effects do they have in the body?

Carbohydrates are used as energy and directly affect the body's hormone balance. When you eat carbohydrates, the body secretes the hormone insulin into the blood to help glucose (sugar) enter the cells, where it is used as energy. If, after a meal, there is more glucose available than the body needs, the insulin instructs the glucose to be stored as glycogen in the liver and the muscles, if there is available room for storage. When the liver and the muscles have filled up their small storehouses, the sugar is converted to fat and is stored in the fat cells where there is sufficient room. Food with a lot of carbohydrates leads to fluctuating blood sugar-levels, and when blood sugar levels decline, hunger and craving for sweets occur, which often leads to eating more high carb foods. This is one of the reasons that relatively sedentary people gain weight on modern diets.

How many carbohydrates do we need?

In principle, we don't need to eat carbohydrates at all, because we can produce enough glucose to cover the cells' needs ourselves. If we don't eat carbohydrates, the body will produce 30–40 grams of glucose daily from components in proteins (amino acids) or fat (glycerol). Instead of imposing this work on the body, you can eat 50–70 grams of carbohydrates each day to make sure you get enough.

Which carbohydrates are sensible to eat?

The best carbohydrate sources are those which are rich in nutrition and provide little increase in blood sugar. These are foods such as vegetables, nuts, berries, fruit, natural yoghurt, cottage cheese, pulses and whole grains. If your carbohydrate consumption is as low as 50 grams per day divided among three meals, it doesn't matter which foods you choose, because the majority of the meals will then consist of fat and proteins, and the blood sugar increase will remain low regardless. If you wish to eat more carbohydrates, you should choose foods that yield the least blood sugar increase, for example, the coarsest breads with a lot of rye and whole grains, wholemeal pasta and brown rice. Beginning on page 217, you'll find more detailed information about my diet recommendations.

What are proteins?

Proteins are large molecules assembled by amino acids. Of the 20 amino acids that are found in the body, eight are essential for adults and nine for small children; in other words, we need to obtain them from our diet because the body cannot create them itself. Proteins which contain all the essential amino acids are called complete proteins. Examples of foods that contain complete protein are meat, poultry, fish, eggs, dairy products and soybeans. Vegetable foods other than soybeans do not contain complete proteins and must therefore be combined. Animal protein is generally better than vegetable protein, but if we eat different vegetable foods in the same meal, the protein quality in the meal will be satisfactory. Good protein sources for vegetarians are nuts, seeds, pulses, soya products, grain products, egg products and dairy products.

What does the body use proteins for, and what effects do they have in the body?

Protein is included in all the body's cells and is important for maintaining normal muscle mass. Sufficient protein consumption reduces muscle loss during weight reduction.

Sufficient protein provides a feeling of fullness, slows down the blood sugar increase in a meal that contains carbohydrates, and increases the release of the hormone glucagon, which stimulates fat metabolism. Protein increases the release of growth hormone, which among other things, stimulates muscle growth. Twenty-five percent of the energy in proteins is converted to heat during the metabolism process and cannot be stored.

The body manages to make use of only a certain quantity

of protein per meal. The quantity depends on body size and activity level.

How much protein do we need?

Proteins build up and maintain hormones, enzymes, muscles, connective tissue and hair, among other things. For this, a daily 0.5–1.5 grams per kilogram of body weight is required, depending on activity level and muscle mass. If you eat a lot of fat, the protein demand is lower because the quantity of enzymes that is required to convert glucose to energy is lower. Muscle mass is very important for an effective metabolism, because muscles burn more energy than fat tissue.

Which proteins are sensible for us to eat?

Good protein sources are fish, shellfish, poultry, meat, eggs, cheese, cottage cheese, nuts and almonds. Nuts and almonds also contain a lot of fat of the type many people get too little of. Take care that the high protein food you eat doesn't contain too many carbohydrates (starch and sugar). Choose pure food as often as possible and avoid mixed products like sausages, saveloy, fish balls, fish cakes, meatballs and ready-to-eat meals. Read the contents when you buy packaged goods, and gradually you'll teach yourself to choose correctly.

What is fat?

Fat is divided into saturated, mono-unsaturated and poly-unsaturated fat. The division is decided by how the fat molecules have been formed. Fat sources contain various quantities of these three fat types.

Animal fat is found in meat, poultry, offal, tallow, lard, fish, shellfish, eggs and dairy products. A little over half of the fatty acids in fat from animals are mono-unsaturated and polyunsaturated fatty acids, except for dairy products, where the proportion is approximately a third. The rest are saturated fats.

Vegetable fat comes from sources such as grain, pulses, nuts, almonds, seeds, olives, avocado, vegetable oils and vegetable margarine.

Vegetable oils are oils extracted from vegetable (plant) sources. Cold-pressed oils have kept most of their original quality and the most nutrients in the extraction process. Hot-pressed oils (also called refined oils) are created by the raw material being heated up and then being pressed and filtered. This process reduces the content of nutrients, changes the taste and damages the fatty acids. Extracted oils, in addition to refining, have chemicals added to make the most of the raw materials, which damages the fatty acids and further reduces the quantity of nutrients and the taste. The most commonly used oils are liquid at room temperature because they are rich in unsaturated and polyunsaturated fatty acids. Oils such as soya oil and sunflower oil contain primarily polyunsaturated fat and are therefore liquid even if they are kept in a refrigerator. Olive oil, on the other hand, congeals a little in the refrigerator because it contains mostly mono-unsaturated fat, some saturated fat and little polyunsaturated fat. Coconut oil contains a lot of saturated fat, is soft at room temperature and becomes hard in the refrigerator. Oils with a lot of polyunsaturated fat should be kept in dark bottles because it reduces the light's negative effect on the oil.

Polyunsaturated fatty acids are divided into omega-3 and omega-6 fatty acids. The two fatty acids alpha-linolenic acid (omega-3) and linoleic acid (omega-6) must be provided via diet because we cannot produce them ourselves. Therefore, they are called the essential fatty acids. Most people get far too many omega-6 fatty acids in relation to omega-3 fatty acids. Therefore, it can be important to increase the consumption of omega-3 and reduce the consumption of omega-6 fatty acids. In some cases, however, the omega-6 fatty acids we get have been so damaged because of heat treatment, exposure to sunlight or rough processing (refining) that we should also provide more of these in natural form.

Researchers have discovered that Stone Age people ate more omega-3 and less omega-6 fatty acids than we do today. The relationship between the two fatty acids in the diet of the past has been estimated at 1–2:1 in favour of omega-6 fatty acids. Today this has been changed considerably. The relationship is considered to be 10–15:1. In the U.S., many people consume 30 times more omega-6 than omega-3 fatty acids. This has great consequences for our health, because, among other things, a large excess of omega-6 fatty acids promotes inflammation. To make the whole thing a little more difficult, there are also some omega-6 fatty acids with omega-3-like properties. To achieve better balance between the essential fatty acids, we should increase the consumption of omega-3 fatty acids and omega-6 fatty acids with omega-3-like properties, reduce the consumption of food products which contain a lot of omega-6 fatty acids, and consume instead a few "fresh" omega-6 fatty acids in the form of nuts, seeds, vegetables and perhaps dietary supplements such as Udo's Choice and evening primrose oil. To make it simple:

this balance will improve greatly if you reduce your consumption of grains and oils that have a lot of omega-6 fatty acids, and eat oily fish, nuts and seeds several times a week.

Some common food products that contain essential fatty acids.

Omega-6 fatty acids we get too much of	Omega-6 fatty acids we get too little of	Omega-3 fatty acids we get too little of
Corn oil	Evening primrose oil	Linseed oil
Sunflower oil	Vegetables	Canola oil
Soya oil	Pulses	Walnut oil
Peanut oil		Vegetables
Grain		Oily fish
		Pulses

Ready-made food often contains a lot of omega-6 fatty acids, often of poor quality, so avoid it as much as possible. If you reduce grain consumption significantly, you will also greatly reduce consumption of these omega-6 fatty acids. Modern producion gives meat that also contains a good deal of omega-6 fatty acids because the animals are grain fed. Wild game, which contains less omega-6 and more omega-3 fatty acids, is more beneficial.

Trans fatty acids are a group of polyunsaturated fatty acids which, with certain exceptions, are not found in nature. They have properties that resemble saturated fatty acids, but synthetic trans fatty acids look a little different from the natural ones. They are created when plant oils are heated up and hydrogen is added artificially. The fat then becomes less liquid, which is how margarine is made. Even though synthetic trans fatty acids resemble saturated fatty acids, they have other biological properties and many unfortunate effects. Studies have shown, among other things, that they contribute to cardiovascular disease and cancer. The most important source of synthetic trans fatty acids in most countries is margarine. Transfats are also often used for deep-frying in the fast food industry, in frozen foods that are breaded, in processed and packaged cakes, buns, biscuits, certain breads, dry soup and sauce mixes, and crisps. The labelling of trans fat in food products is often poor. On some packages, hydrogenated or partially hydrogenated vegetable fat appears, and these products can contain trans fat. In addition, they contain other unnatural combinations and residues.

What does the body use fat for, and what effects does it have on the body?

Fat has many important functions in the body and is vital for the formation of every single tiny cell. Fat constitutes an important part of all cell membranes and serves as insulation against the cold, protects sensitive organs and is a primary component of the brain. Fat is the body's most important form of energy storage, and fatty acids are consequently the body's most important energy source. The body stores fat in the form of triglycerides which consist of three fatty acids and one glycerol molecule.

Strange as it may sound, for someone who wants to lose weight, it is important to have fat for every meal. The less fat we eat, the worse the body becomes at burning fat. Fat in food stimulates fat metabolism and increases neither blood sugar nor the secretion of insulin.

How much fat do we need?

Nutritional authorities in the Western world advise that fat should not account for more then 30-35 % of the energy we receive from our food. No one, however, goes around and calculates this every day. If you eat low fat dairy products, lean meat and lean fish, you may reach the target. But what is the point of that? A high consumption of natural fat is not dangerous if you simultaneously restrict the consumption of carbohydrates substantially. It is, however, detrimental to eat a lot of processed fat in combination with a lot of carbohydrates. If, on the other hand, you reduce your consumption of carbohydrates, you should eat more natural fat. You are then using mostly fat as an energy source instead of glucose from food products containing sugar and starch (fruit, juice, bread, cereal, potatoes, pasta, rice).

How much fat you need depends on your gender, age, weight and how active you are. It regulates itself as a rule, for there are limits to how much fat you'll manage to eat when you don't combine it with carbohydrates. Sugar makes fat taste better and simultaneously stimulates the appetite, so that we overeat more easily than when we only eat fat. Most people will quickly feel full and unwell if they eat a lot of fat by itself.

What type of fat is it sensible to eat?

I advise you to eat natural fat whenever possible; that found in meat, oily fish, chicken with the skin on, fatty poultry (goose and duck), nuts, almonds, seeds, avocado, olives, butter, cream, sour cream, crème fraîche, rich cheese, cold-pressed olive oil, canola oil, linseed oil and coconut oil.

Overweight and obesity

Overweight and obesity epidemic

The World Health Organization (WHO) has defined criteria for what is underweight, normal weight, overweight and obese. You can see the definitions for adults over 18 years in the table below. BMI is an abbreviation for body mass index. You can figure out your BMI by taking your weight, measured in kilograms and dividing it by your height (in metres*) squared.

Metric	Imperial
90 kg and 1.7 m	200 lb x .45 = 90 kg
$(1.7 \times 1.7) = 1.7^2 = 2.89$	$(5 \text{ ft} \times .305) + (7 \text{ in} \times .025) = 1.7 \text{ m}$
BMI = 90/2.89 = 31	

If you have trouble calculating your BMI, you can go online to find many convenient BMI-calculators.

BMI says nothing about the composition of the body, so for weight lifters and others with large amounts of muscle mass this measurement is of little use. Muscular people can have a BMI over 25 even though they have low body fat. To find out the body composition, one must use special equipment that gives muscle mass and fat in weight and percentages. However, for the great majority of us, BMI is still a handy measurement to relate to.

* 1 lb ≈ .45 kg / 1 ft ≈ .305 m / 1 in ≈ .025 m

Designation	BMI (kg/m2)
Underweight	< 18.5
Normal weight	18.5–24.9
Overweight	25–29.9
Obese	Grade 1: 30–34.9
	Grade 2: 35–39.9
	Grade 3: > 40

In Norway, people who have a BMI over 40, or over 35 with additional health problems, are defined as being chronically ill. These people have the right to public health care. Health surveys show that the average body weight of Norwegians has increased steadily in the last few decades, and this increase applies to all ages and groups. Men in their 40s now weigh on average 5 kilograms (11 pounds) more, while women in the same age group weigh 5.8 kilograms (12.8 pounds) more than just 15 years ago.

In 2008, a large health survey was carried out in Norway of 3511 students aged 8–9 years old. The survey showed the following:

- 14 % of the girls were overweight, and additionally 4 % were obese
- 12 % of the boys were overweight, and additionaly 3.5 % were obese

The fact that more children are becoming overweight and obese will probably lead to a further increase in the percentage of adults who are overweight and obese.

Gunnhild had put on a lot of weight and wanted to lose it

Gunnhild was approaching 40 and was tired of being overweight. After years of back problems and a back operation, her physical activity had become limited. Her weight increased steadily, and there were more spare tyres around her waist. Several other members of the family were overweight. Two of them had type 1 diabetes, while her mother's mother had been diagnosed with type 2 diabetes. Gunnhild never had any serious illnesses apart from back problems and used no medication. The last few years she had, however, developed various symptoms that bothered her. When she ate foods like bread, buns and pasta, she often got hyperacidity and cramps in her stomach. Eating grain products also led to loose stools many times a day. Also, her legs had become very swollen, and the rings on her fingers had started to tighten. Gunnhild thought she was eating sensibly, since she stuck to coarse bread, lots of vegetables and five fruits a day. As a rule she ate sweets only at parties and now and then when she was alone. Her weight was 102.6 kilograms (16 stone 2), her BMI 37 and her blood pressure 140/90 mm Hg.

I explained to Gunnhild that a great many people have stomach problems from grain products, and that I figured that the problems would disappear if she cut out foods made from flour. She was surprised when I said that five fruits a day was not healthy for her because fruit contains a lot of sugar. She had, of course, heard about "five a day" and thought she was being smart to follow the advice. We agreed that she would, over the course of a week or two, gradually remove foods which contained sugar and starch, so that she was left with a total of 20–30 grams per day (ketogenic diet, see page 229). I said that she had to replace the carbohydrates with natural fat and a little more protein. She thought this sounded very strange, because it went against what she had previously learned about what a sensible diet is composed of. I said, "You've followed the official guidelines for years now, and yet you're still putting on weight. Since you're seeking my advice, I think you have to try this – it can't hurt to try it for a couple of months and see what happens." She was willing to do so but looked rather disconcerted when she left the office.

Gunnhild returned after four weeks and said that she had read the information I had given her. She had a strong desire to lose weight, so she had started the ketogenic diet the day after she'd been to see me. A few days later she had been a little dizzy and had a headache, but that had quickly passed. Her stomach was functioning very well, she had a normal bowel movement every day and was pain-free after meals. She also felt that she had far more energy and didn't need her afternoon nap any longer. Her weight was 6 kilograms (13 pounds) lower after four weeks, and she was extremely pleased. Convinced that this was the right diet for her, her motivation increased gradually as she watched the weight fall off.

The blood samples she had taken the day after our first consultation showed that her levels of C-peptide, ALAT, and gamma GT were too high and that her levels of SHBG and vitamin D were too low (see page 280, 285, 288 and 289). I explained to her that all the values would normalise if she continued with the new diet and took vitamin D supplements.

Gunnhild returned after six weeks. Christmas was behind

us, and she had lost another 3 kilograms (6.5 pounds). She had managed Christmas quite well; she'd enjoyed a little fruit and low-sugar marzipan. The most difficult part had been what to say when she was offered cakes, desserts and chocolates at parties. We discussed different strategies and arrived at the conclusion that she could take along nuts and 70 percent chocolate when she was going to a party. Also, she could quite simply say to family and friends that she had prediabetes and couldn't eat sweets because of her blood sugar. Most people accept this, so it's often smarter than saying that you're dieting.

After another four weeks, Gunnhild had reduced her weight by another 3 kilograms (6.5 pounds), but had lost a little of her appetite. So I gave her recipes for protein bread and pancakes containing only a few carbohydrates, and redommendations for low carb cookbooks. I showed her how few carbohydrates there are in a portion of raspberries and cream and suggested that she should eat berries every day with an unsweetened dairy product, for example, cottage cheese or cream, and/or nuts. She thought bran bread was also a handy alternative at times when she needed something to munch on. New blood tests were ordered, and Gunnhild was very eager to know if there were any improvements.

After four months, Gunnhild was 16 kilograms (2 stone 7) lighter, and all the blood test values were normal. Gunnhild was extremely pleased and felt that she now had enough knowledge to continue losing weight on her own. I asked her to come back if she got on the wrong track again.

Blood test results before and after diet change.

Blood test	Before	After 3 months	Reference range
C-peptide (pmol/L)	1452	592	< 700
SHBG (nmol/L)	14	31	23–100
ALAT (U/L)	75	31	8–46
Gamma GT (U/L)	53	29	10–42
Vitamin D3 (nmol/L)	41	70	50–150

Excessive level of C-peptide

C-peptide is an expression for the production of the hormone insulin in the pancreas. If the cells are insensitive (resistant) to insulin, there has to be more insulin in order for this hormone to have any effect. Insulin has, among other things, the task of opening the cell walls so that glucose can be transported into the cells. A high C-peptide value thus means that you are insulin resistant, something which means that you easily put on weight because insulin stimulates fat storage and inhibits fat metabolism.

Low levels of SHBG
(sexual hormone binding globulin)

SHBG is often low in the case of polycystic ovary syndrome (PCOS), which is discussed on pages 179–191. However, I just as often find low values among women who do not have PCOS, but who do have a high insulin level. It is insulin that is the reason for SHBG being low, and this results in an increased quantity of active testosterone in the blood among women.

Excessive levels of ALAT and gamma GT (liver tests)

Insulin inhibits fat metabolism, so when insulin levels are elevated, less fat is being used for energy. Moreover, insulin stimulates fat storage, and therefore fat is created from glucose in the liver and in the fat cells. This is why consuming a lot of carbohydrates and high insulin levels result in the accumulation of fat in the liver. With fatty liver syndrome one often sees elevated liver values, which has been shown in many studies. The table on the preceding page shows that the liver function test values are normalised with weight reduction on a low carb diet.

Insufficient level of vitamin D

Studies show that a relatively large share of Norwegians have low levels of vitamin D in the blood, especially during winter. People who are overweight, insulin resistant and diabetic very often have low values. The concentration of vitamin D can be checked with a common blood test (1.25-OH-vitamin D_3), and if the level is low, I recommend a supplement and another blood test after a while.

Causes of obesity

Obesity is now regarded as a chronic disease caused by a complex interplay of hereditary and environmental factors. Researchers think that approximately 50 percent of all obesity is hereditary. I think this is a somewhat strange way of looking at it. If there is something we inherit, it is the characteristic that we put on weight when we eat too many carbohydrates. In addition, there is something called epigenetic inheritance, which deals with how food or other substances we consume via air and water override our genes so that they change their behavior. This means that the genes are controlled by, for example, the food we eat and are not then necessarily our "fate".

Let me compare humans with grizzly bears, who put on weight heavily in the autumn. The grizzly bear is a meat and plant eater like us. When it comes out of it's den in spring, it is slim and lives off roots, tubers, fish, rodents, deer and grazing animals. When the berries are ripe in autumn, it's time to put on weight in order to get itself through the winter. And what is it that gives the bear's body the signal to gain weight? Indeed, it is sugar and, consequently, the production of insulin, exactly as with humans. The bear eats enormous quantities of berries, increases one third of its body weight, and in this way it can survive until spring on its own body fat.

Stone Age people found themselves in a similar situation. Winter was cold, and food was limited to meat, birds and fish. In the summer, however, they found carbohydrates in the form of vegetables, fruit, berries and nuts, which helped them put on fat for winter use. Some people gain weight from carbohydrates more readily than others. People with these genes will do better in periods when food is scarce. The problem today is that we get too many carbohydrates, which results in these people gaining weight rapidly. The simple message therefore is that people who gain weight easily should approximate a Stone Age diet in order to keep themselves slim and healthy.

A common cause of overweight and obesity is synthetic medicine. Examples of these are cortisone and medications that are used to treat epilepsy and mental disorders. It is not yet clear how these medicines work in relation to obesity, but in my experience, patients who use medicines for epilepsy and mental disorders manage to lose weight on a strict low carb diet. Many have experienced gaining 20–30 kilograms (40–60 pounds) in a short time when they use cortisone tablets. This is because cortisone increases blood sugar by breaking down proteins. Consequently, the insulin level increases, stimulating fat storage and inhibiting fat metabolism. Reducing weight during ongoing cortisone treatment goes, therefore, more slowly than otherwise.

Psychological factors are also important with weight gain. It's not uncommon to use carbohydrates to get into a better mood or to suppress anger, unease and anxiety. If you recognise yourself in this, think about what you eat when you are feeling low and eat for comfort. It's probably not beef or salmon. Perhaps you eat chocolate, potato crisps, cakes, fruit – or bread, if you don't have anything else? The problem is that these carbohydrates only provide a short term good feeling, and you have to eat more when your blood sugar drops again about an hour later.

Sugar, insulin and obesity

Our blood sugar level varies considerably after meals, depending on the food we eat. In the figure on the next page, you will see how the level varies after twenty healthy people consumed five different test meals with varying carbohydrate content. As you see, there is a large increase in blood sugar after eating a high carbohydrate meal, and almost no changes after eating chicken.

Insulin is a hormone that is produced in the pancreas. It is an energy and fat storage hormone that is responsible for blood sugar not becoming too high, and which, among other things, results in increased production of fatty acids, increased levels of triglycerides (fat) in the blood and in-

Concentration of glucose in the blood (serum blood glucose) after consumption of five test meals of 60 grams.
(HC = high carbohydrate meal; WB = white bread;
MC = moderate carbohydrate meal; LC = low carbohydrate meal; CH = chicken.)

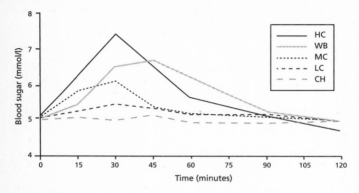

Source: Hertzler SR, Kim Y. Glycemic and insulenemic response to energy bars of differing macronutrient composition in healthy adults. Medical Science Monitor 2003;9:CR84-90.

creased uptake of free fatty acids in fatty tissue. Insulin opens the cell walls so that glucose from the blood can be transported into the cells. Glucose is either used there as energy or is stored as glycogen in the liver and muscles and as fat in fatty tissue. In addition, insulin inhibits fat metabolism. If you eat a lot of carbohydrates, you will produce a lot of insulin. Conversely, if you eat few carbohydrates, you will produce little insulin. In the next diagram, you can see how the concentration of insulin in the blood varies when twenty healthy people consume five different meals composed of different carbohydrates. It is obvious that there is a large increase in insulin after consuming a high carb meal and

Concentration of insulin in the blood (serum insulin response) after consumption of five test meals of 60 grams. (HC = high carbohydrate meal; WB = white bread; MC = moderate carbohydrate meal; LC = low carbohydrate meal; CH = chicken.)

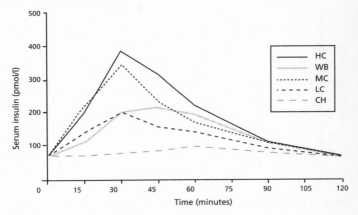

Source: Hertzler SR, Kim Y. Glycemic and insulenemic response to energy bars of differing macronutrient composition in healthy adults. Medical Science Monitor 2003;9:CR84-90.

white bread, while the curve is nearly flat after eating of chicken.

Insulin resistance

A body becomes resistant to insulin when its ability to use glucose in a suitable manner is impaired. The liver and muscle cells become less sensitive to insulin. In other words, they no longer open as easily when the insulin gives the signal that they should open up to absorb glucose. The body tries to compensate by producing more insulin, which only leads to further insulin resistance. The fat cells, however, remain sensitive to insulin, so that glucose is converted to fat and is stored in the fatty tissue instead. The body can control blood sugar in this way for many years, but the flip side is weight gain. Finally, the fat cells become insulin resistant as well, and then the weight no longer increases. There are many degrees of insulin resistance, but in reality, type 2 diabetes is fully developed insulin resistance. The cause of insulin resistance is principally too many carbohydrates in the diet over a long period. This leads to elevated insulin levels, first in connection with meals, and eventually during the night as well. Insulin resistance is developed as a countermeasure to too much sugar and insulin. The body quite simply doesn't tolerate all the sugar and protects itself by becoming insensitive to insulin. Some people have lower tolerance for carbohydrates than others and develop insulin resistance, even though they haven't eaten any differently than other people they know, who are not insulin resistant. The genes we inherit from our parents and grandparents determine whether we are predisposed to insulin resistance, while our own lifestyle determines whether or when we develop it.

The body can be insulin resistant for many years before diabetes develops. During this period, it is very easy to gain weight, because the whole time there are massive amounts of insulin present, instructing the body to store energy and turn off its fat metabolism. At this point, you are caught in a vicious cycle and you put on weight even though you're not eating a lot. You've become an efficient "fat storage machine." The fat is often added around the stomach, and you get an "apple shape". This stomach fat is the dangerous fat that leads to an increased risk of clogged arteries and heart attack.

The production of insulin in the pancreas begins with the

formation of a long amino acid called proinsulin. It is split into one molecule of insulin and one molecule of C-peptide.

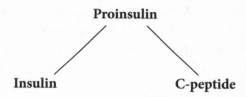

Insulin is the biologically active hormone, but because of a relatively long half-life in the blood, the concentration of C-peptide is a better measure of insulin secretion than the concentration of insulin. Up until 2004, the reference range for C-peptide (fasting) at the hormone laboratory at the former Aker University Hospital (now Oslo University Hospital, Aker) was 240–720 pmol/L. In 2004, the reference range was changed to 220–1400 pmol/L. The new reference range is not due to a change in method but reflects, instead, an increased insulin production in the population. In the laboratory's analysis handbook it says, "There is reason to believe that patients who have an insulin concentration in the upper half of the reference range are insulin resistant, which can have implications for their lipid profile, blood pressure and cardiovascular risk (the metabolic risk syndrome)." My impression is that most doctors are not familiar with this, so don't react to C-peptide values that are under 1400 pmol/L. I use 700 pmol/L as the upper limit, which indicate in parentheses behind the actual value in the patient history. What the optimal level is for C-peptide, we do not know.

Studies have shown that chronically high insulin levels,

from either injections or production by the pancreas, leads to insulin resistance. A person with type 1 diabetes can become insulin resistant from consuming a lot of carbohydrates and subsequently using a lot of insulin. This leads to the need for even higher doses of insulin to keep the blood sugar under control. The result is often overweight, in the same way as people who produce a lot of insulin on their own.

The most important debilitating effects of a chronically elevated sugar and insulin level:

- Promotes inflammation in the body and thus contributes, to muscle and joint pain, arteriosclerosis and heart disease.
- Increases excretion of magnesium via the kidneys, which can lead to leg cramps, migraine, high blood pressure and increased risk of heart disease.
- Reduces release of nitrogen oxide (NO), which contributes to increased blood pressure.
- Hinders excretion of sodium (salt), which leads to water accumulating in the body and contributes to high blood pressure.
- Leads to blood platelets sticking together and consequently to the formation of blood clots.
- Can cause kidney damage, lead to impotence and cause damage to the eyes, because the blood supply is being obstructed by constriction of, and damage to, small blood vessels.
- Increases the risk of many different forms of cancer.
- Leads to increased formation of triglycerides (fat) and cholesterol.

- Causes intermitant drops in blood sugar, which is associated with a range of physical and mental problems.
- Leads to obesity from increased storage of fat in the fat cells and blocked fat metabolism.
- Increases the risk of type 2 diabetes because the liver and muscle cells, and eventually the fat cells, become less sensitive to the effects of insulin.
- Leads to a hormonal imbalance in men by reducing the formation of testosterone and increasing the production of cortisol (stress hormone).
- Leads to a hormonal imbalance in women because estrogen production becomes continuously high instead of cyclic and the production of testosterone and cortisol increases.
- Increases the risk of Alzheimer's disease and dementia.
- Reduces the excretion of uric acid, which can result in a high level of uric acid in the blood and potentially gout.

Rita weighed 265 kilograms (41 stone 10) at 25 years old

Rita came to me because she wanted to lose weight. She had her entire patient journal with her, which I read. At seven years of age, she was referred to a paediatrician because she was 18 kilograms (2 stone 12) overweight. She was monitored and weighed regularly by a public health nurse throughout her entire childhood. Her parents were told that it was just "puppy fat" that she would grow out of. At school, she was bullied a lot because she was so big and her clothes weren't fashionable. Rita had a difficult time and felt extremely lonesome. At 16, she was examined by a specialist in hormone diseases at a local hospital. She was then 175 centimetres (5 feet 9 inches) tall, weighed 138 kilograms (21 stone 10), her menstruation was irregular, she had a buffalo hump (fat accumulation on the neck) and blue stretch marks on her chest and back. Blood tests showed that she had significant insulin resistance, while other blood tests and examinations were normal. Treatment with metformin was started, which can improve insulin sensitivity and reduce the production of sugar in the liver, though it had no effect on Rita's weight. She then met with a nutritionist, who recommended a standard reduced fat diet with lots of carbohydrates in the form of coarse bread, potatoes, rice, pasta, vegetables and fruit.

When Rita was 19 years old, she weighed 145 kilograms (22 stone 12), was plagued with pains in her knees and had problems moving normally. She was treated with Xenical, which reduces the uptake of fat in the intestine, and Reductil, which can inhibit appetite – without there being any noteworthy effect on her weight.

At 21, Rita weighed over 200 kilograms (31 stone 7) and was again referred to a nutritionist, where she got the same advice as before. She was granted disability benefits and had a check-up with her regular doctor every month. In 2002, Rita sought patient injury compensation because she had gained weight even though she followed the dietary advice. Her application was denied on the grounds that she had been well-examined and monitored and that no disease could be established that explained the overweight problem. Her general practioner (GP) eventually recommended a gastric bypass operation, but with a weight of 240 kilograms (37 stone 11), she didn't dare go through with such an operation. In 2004, she had several conversations with psychiatrists in the hope that it might influence her to want the gastric bypass operation. This did not succeed, and Rita was again referred several times to the medical ward at the hospital because the GP felt it was difficult to bear the responsibility for her obesity alone. The feedback from the medical ward was that they had nothing to offer for obesity beyond excluding hormonal disease.

Rita mostly stayed indoors. It was difficult to walk, and she tired with the slightest exertion. In the summer, she sat constantly in front of a table fan to avoid the heat, but she struggled nonetheless with hot flushes and breathing difficulties. In the winter, she went without a winter jacket because it was impossible to find one that was large enough. On the coldest days, her arms and shoulders were purple after being out for a short walk. She weighed 265 kilograms (41 stone 10) when she was 25 years old, and health personnel said that she wasn't likely to see her 30th birthday. Her father was distraught over his daughter's weight problems. He tied her in place in the car with a rope (the safety belt was too small), and drove her over 500 kilometres (300 miles) to Oslo in the hope of getting help.

At the first consultation, Rita said that she had eaten an ordinary Norwegian diet which she had been given at home. She had not eaten a lot of sweets, cakes, potato crisps or the like, and said that even though she had followed the dietary advice she received, she had still gained weight. Rita trained with a physiotherapist three times a week, an hour at a time. She used no medication but took two cod liver oil capsules each day. The last weight measurement using two scales at the GP's office showed approximately 265 kilograms (41 stone 10), while her BMI was calculated at 85.

Because Rita lived far from Oslo, we agreed that in the future she would weigh herself at her GP's office. The blood samples that were taken from her after the first consultation showed sky-high values for insulin production (C-peptide and insulin). Her fasting blood sugar level was normal (4.3 mmol/L), but the long-term blood sugar was a little high. The level of folate (vitamin B) was too low, and the values for uric acid, Micro-CRP and ferritin were too high (see page 290, 285, 283 and 284). Rita wanted to start with a VLCD (very low calorie diet. See page 232), which is a powder diet with few carbohydrates and calories but with sufficient proteins and fat. She started with five products and lots of low carb vegetables and took supplements of salts, vitamins and omega-3 fatty acids. Further consultations were conducted by telephone.

Rita had consulted with her GP bi-weekly for a long time and continued with this. The first 15 days she lost 17 kilograms (2 stone 9). She liked the VLCD products but was very nauseous after every meal. She didn't want to continue with this diet and was instead recommended the ketogenic diet with a daily consumption of approximately 20 grams of carbohydrates but no limit of calories. Information about this diet was given over the telephone, and afterwards she received written material. Based on this, she made a personal menu plan. I allowed her to send me text messages freely, which she did frequently. In this way, she received frequent advice, support and encouragement.

On the first telephone consultation after that summer, she had lost 75 kilograms (11 stone 11) in two months, and we agreed that she could start with one piece of fruit every day because she missed it. Eventually, she also introduced one Yoplait yogurt daily. After three months, she had reduced her weight by 93 kilograms (14 stone 9) and at this point she included a small carrot each day.

A simple arithmetic equation of Rita's energy intake

shows the following: The daily energy requirement is about 265 kilograms x 30 kcal/kilogram = 8000 kcal (584 pounds x 13.7 kcal/pound = 8000 kcal). In other words, she had a daily energy requirement of approximately 8000 kcal for maintenance, and so that she could manage to move her large body. When she ate the recommended high carb, low fat diet of approximately 2000 kcal, she had a daily deficiency of approximately 6000 kcal, and in principle should have lost nearly one kilogram (two pounds) daily (7000 kcal represents approximately one kilogram (two pounds) of fat). Instead, her weight increased by approximately one kilogram (two pounds) a month. When she ate the ketogenic diet with about the same amount of energy, it corresponded better with arithmetic equation, because her weight was then reduced by 93 kilograms (14 stone 9) in 90 days.

The weight loss stabilised itself gradually at approximately one kilogram (two pounds) per week after the introduction of a few more carbohydrates. Rita thought this rate of weight loss was sufficient because such great changes were happening to her body. She was monitored via monthly telephone consultations and frequent SMS contact. A general blood test was taken every third month to follow the development. She felt good the entire time she was on the diet and was eventually able to expand her physical activities considerably. She started to go on daily walks which were gradually increased to six miles per day. Eventually Rita could buy her clothes in regular shops. She wept with joy the first time she bought herself a smart pair of slacks and a tunic.

After two years, she returned for a consultation. She then weighed 97 kilograms (15 stone 4) and was unrecognisable after having reduced her weight by 168 kilograms (26 stone

6). She was 177 centimetres (5 feet 10 inches) tall, and a body fat scale showed the following: fat mass 32 kilograms (5 stone 1), muscle mass 62 kilograms (9 stone 11) and BMI 31.

Rita's fat mass after two years was only one kilogram (two pounds) over the upper normal value. She had a fat mass that was about normal, but her muscle mass and extra skin contributed significantly to the weight of 97 kilograms (15 stone 4). She had developed strong muscles from carrying such a heavy body for many years. Rita is now waiting for plastic surgery to remove the excess skin. All her blood tests are normal. She dreams of having a husband, children, her own house and car; things most people her age take for granted. Rita has an education she hasn't used but is now in a full-time job and glad to be doing something socially useful.

Blood test results before and after diet change.

Blood test	Before	After 2 years	Reference range
Long-term blood sugar (%)	6.1	4.8	< 6.1
C-peptide (pmol/L)	3939	676	< 700
Insulin (pmol/L)	667	29	< 120
Folate (nmol/L)	4.9	36.6	> 5.7
Micro-CRP (mg/L)	>20	1.3	< 5
Ferritin (µg/L)	206	42	15–200
Uric acid (µmol/L)	479	285	155–350

Excessive long-term blood sugar

When fasting blood sugar is normal and long-term blood sugar is too high, it means that the blood sugar has been elevated after meals, so that the average blood sugar remains high. This blood test says something about what the blood sugar has been the last six to eight weeks before the samples were taken.

Excessive insulin levels

Insulin is a term for the production of the hormone insuline in the pancreas, as is C-peptide. The high level in this case indicates insulin resistance. The value can also be high in those who inject insulin.

Insufficient level of folate (vitamin B)

As a rule, this is due to having too little folate in the diet or reduced uptake in the intestine.

Excessive level of CRP and ferritin – chronic inflammation

With a large fat mass, a great deal of inflammation develops. The degree of inflammation can be measured by various blood tests, such as CRP. Elevated CRP is a risk factor for cardiovascular disease, but not the cause of it. Studies have shown that CRP is reduced much more by low carb diets than by low fat/high carb diets. Ferritin is also often released into the blood in large quantities with inflammation. As you can see from the table above, CRP and ferritin were considerably lower after normalising insulin production and the large weight loss.

Excessive level of uric acid

Studies have shown that insulin inhibits the excretion of uric acid in the kidneys, and my experience is that a great many people with high insulin production have a lot of uric acid in the blood. The value is normalised on a low carb diet because the insulin level is reduced.

Traditional treatment of overweight and obesity – does it work?

The usual advice, which you are surely familiar with, is based on reducing the energy content of our food, for example, by about 500 kcal per day. Theoretically this can yield a weight loss of approximately 0.5 kilograms (1 pound) per week because 7000 kcal represents approximately one kilogram (two pounds) of fat. But this is only theoretical, because humans quite simply do not function quite like an oven – which has been the model until now!

To find out how much energy the various nutrients contain, researchers use a type of oven (bomb calorimeter) to measure how much energy is created in the form of heat. In this way, it has been calculated that 1 gram of protein and 1 gram of carbohydrate contain approximately 4 kcal, while 1 gram of alcohol contains 7 kcal and 1 gram of fat, 9 kcal. Fat contains the most energy, and that is why all dieters have learnt that they have to eat a low fat diet. But our body is so much more complicated than this. Proteins, fat, carbohydrates and alcohol have vastly different hormonal effects in the body, which is critical for metabolism. In other words, it is important to think of where the calories come from, not just how many you eat.

Typical official Dietary Advice

1. Eat *at least* three portions of vegetables and two portions of fruit daily.
2. Choose boiled or baked potatoes instead of crisps and chips.
3. Eat coarse grain and bread products.

4. Eat more fish – both as a spread and for dinner.
5. Choose lean meat and dairy products.
6. Choose soft vegetable margarine or oil instead of hard margarine or butter.
7. Cut down on the consumption of sugar, especially in the form of soda and sweets.
8. Be careful with salt.
9. Water is best for quenching thirst.

Furthermore, you are advised that 30 minutes' daily physical activity is beneficial.

Comments on the above advice

Some people can eat this type of food and stay slim. How healthy they remain is, however, another matter. My experience is that many people put on weight from this type of high carb diet. And once you've become heavy and insulin resistant, it's nearly impossible to achieve a normal weight again on this diet. One must, in any case, have an iron will and be able to suppress the body's need for more food.

1. Fruit contains a lot of sugar and comes in addition to other sugary and starchy food. Two medium-sized apples contain approximately 30 grams of sugar, and if you eat a banana instead and 100 grams of grapes, you'll get approximately 40 grams of sugar. If you eat five fruits a day, the sugar consumption from fruit quickly adds up to 80–90 grams. If the vegetables you eat are root vegetables, you'll get a rich supply of sugar from these sources as well. Vegetables which grow above ground contain, however, relatively little sugar and can be eaten in large quantities.
2. Boiled or baked potatoes are not necessarily better than

crisps and chips, except if the last two are fried in very unhealthy fat. If you use saturated fat for frying (it tolerates high heat the best), "fat-saturated" crisps provide less blood sugar increase than a boiled potato and, consequently, have less effect on the insulin level in the body. Potatoes contain a great deal of starch, which actually only consists of glucose molecules. If you eat potatoes without fat, you'll get a higher blood sugar than if you eat potatoes with fat. Therefore, it's better to eat some potato and put fat on it. This assumes that you have a low daily consumption of carbohydrates (for example, 50 grams), because the combination of a lot of carbohydrates and a lot of fat is detrimental. People with diabetes and who are overweight should not eat many potatoes at all because of the high content of carbohydrates.

3. Coarse-grained breads are not as coarse as they appear. Often, they have been coloured to look coarse. Genuinely coarse-grained bread is made of 100 percent coarsley ground flour and contains preferably whole grains. Coarse bread doesn't provide as great an increase in blood sugar as white bread but does contain just as much starch, which gives you an abundance of glucose. Coarsely-ground grain is also a double-edged sword because bran hinders the uptake of some important vitamins and minerals.

4. Fish is definitely good to eat, especially oily fish, which gives us lots of beneficial omega-3 fatty acids. Fish fingers, fish cakes and fish balls are not to be recommended, because they contain a lot of starch if they have flour added. To find the best kind, you have to read the ingredients list to see how many carbohydrates there are in the product. As a general rule, the cheaper the product is, the more starch it contains.

5. Lean meat and dairy products are often more expensive than those which contain more fat. Moreover, you don't get as full from the lean kinds and therefore you usually eat larger portions. Fatty dairy products generally taste better than low fat ones – and it's not just me who thinks so! Also, low fat dairy products often contain more sugar than the fatty ones, because the fat is usually replaced with carbohydrates in various forms. Next time you're in a shop, read the ingredients list for premium ice cream and compare it with the ingredients list for light ice cream. Skimmed milk does not have extra starch added; the fat has beeen removed is all. But remember that a litre of skimmed milk contains about 50 grams of lactose. The rest is water, a little protein, and some minerals and vitamins. There are not very many fat-soluble vitamins in skimmed milk, because they were also removed with the fat. Therefore, vitamin D is added to some types of milk so that the population doesn't get a vitamin D deficiency. If you drink 200 ml (8 fluid ounces) of skimmed milk, you'll get about 10 grams (12 grams) of lactose and a greater blood sugar increase than if you drink 200 ml (8 fluid ounces) of full-fat milk. The reason is that the fat in the full-fat milk causes the stomach to be emptied more slowly, and thus the lactose enters more slowly into the small intestine, where it is split into glucose and galactose. Consequently, the blood sugar doesn't increase as rapidly. Furthermore, you feel more full from full-fat milk, so you don't need to snack during the day. A doctoral dissertation from Sweden shows that children who drink full-fat milk regularly have a lower BMI compared to children who seldom or never drink milk. In addition, several studies which show that people who drink full-fat milk have

lower risk of getting cardiovascular disease than those who drink skimmed milk. Right up until 50 years ago, it was claimed that fatty meat and dairy products tasted best and were the most nutritious. If you look in cookbooks from your great grandmother's time, you'll see how they ate: "Take 10 eggs, 1 litre of cream . . . " and so forth.

6. Margarine is unhealthy because the oils from which it is made have undergone several dozen processes with heat and chemicals to get a margarine in hard form. This is not particularly healthy. Butter, on the other hand, is made from natural cream that has been churned and had salt added. We used natural butter for centuries before heart attacks started spreading around the world. The number of heart attacks increased in step with the fact that we steadily ate more margarine that contained synthetic trans fatty acids. This does not prove that margarine causes heart attacks, but there are certain factors which indicate it. Butter is soft at room temperature, and it keeps well until you have used up the package if you use it daily. If you prefer butter that stays soft in the refrigerator, I recommend you blend room temperature butter with a cold-pressed oil to the desired consistency – then, at least, you know what the butter contains. Olive oil and canola oil contain a lot of mono-unsaturated fat and are fine if you don't use too much heat. Oils such as sunflower oil, corn oil and soya oils are not healthy, for they contain a lot of omega-6 fatty acids and don't tolerate heat very well. Getting some unsaturated fatty acids is good for us. We can get them from eating nuts and seeds, but quantities can quickly become too much the way these oils are used today. We use them when we make food at home, but they are also used in large quantities in, for example, industri-

ally-produced bread, cakes, biscuits and prepared food. In this way we get far too many omega-6 fatty acids, which promote inflammatory conditions in the body among other things. Naturally-produced coconut oil is much better, even though it contains over 90 percent saturated fat. Coconut oil tolerates high heat and contains many beneficial fatty acids. Many people use coconut fat in cooking or quite simply as a dietary supplement.

7. Authorities say that a maximum of 10 percent of the energy in a food can come from added sugar, and that's about 10 percent too much. This is, in fact, in addition to the sugar we get via fruit, milk, juice and the starch we get through grain products and potatoes that become sugar in the body. A good alternative to granulated sugar is the natural sugar alcohol erythritol.

8. Salt in moderate amounts is not dangerous if the kidneys are functioning as they should. The problem for some people is that their kidneys do a poor job of excreting sodium, and that can create problems such as water retention and high blood pressure. It has, in fact, been shown that insulin inhibits the excretion of salt through the kidneys. In other words, it is sensible to reduce the consumption of salt for people who are overweight and produce too much insulin, but it's even smarter to reduce the consumption of sugar and starchy foods because then the insulin level will fall, and the kidneys will excrete more salt.

9. Most people agree that pure water is the healthiest way to quench your thirst – and I am no different!

Daily physical activity is always beneficial – unless you're so heavy that you inflict injuries on yourself during the activity.

In that case, it's better to lose weight by dieting first, and then start to exercise.

Weight loss pills and weight loss operations

In the last few years various weight loss pills have come onto the market, and many people have tried these without effects worth mentioning. Patients as young as 13 years old are now being offered weight loss operations, and the number of operations carried out increases every year. The operation carries a certain risk during the surgery itself and can sometimes lead to problems afterwards. For some people, this looks like the only way out – often because they have not tried a low carb diet!

Perpetual dieters

Most overweight people have tried high carb, low fat, low calorie diets many times, only to discover that they quickly put on the weight again and usually end up weighing more than they did before starting the diet. They think that something is wrong with their metabolism. Many discover that they don't lose any weight on such diets, and some even gain weight. What may have worked before no longer does with increasing age and weight. Dieters are often suspected of not adhering to the diet since they don't lose weight.They feel that they don't have control over their bodies and that they gain weight regardless of what they do. My experience is that these people have an intense desire to lose weight and that they can be unbelievably strong-willed when they are on a diet. They can't be blamed for not trying! But, of course, if the diet doesn't work, it feels meaningless to continue. People on low calorie, high carb diets will feel hungry much of the time, and there are limits to how long one can take feeling hungry. It requires immense willpower to carry out such a diet. Some do manage it, but only with enormous effort – and even then they often gain weight again after the diet is over.

My experience is that overweight people find it easier to be on a low carbohydrate diet because they don't have hungerpangs. To be sure, they must avoid some foods which ordinarily have been part of their daily diet, but most think it's worth it. Experience shows that people with insulin resistance must live on a low carbohydrate diet for the rest of their lives, or they will quickly gain weight again.

Tomas was concerned about being overweight

Tomas was 25 years old when he discovered that he had to change his lifestyle. Several people in the family and two of his colleagues at work suffered heart attacks. Tomas's weight had increased steadily from the age of 20, and he had begun to feel concerned. He wanted help with choosing the right food and managing his lifestyle project.

Tomas was a passive member of a fitness club and walked a couple of times a week. His job was stressful, and he was always travelling. He ate a lot of bread and potatoes, and in the evening he snacked on sweets because he had a strong sweet tooth. He drank a lot of Diet Coke and coffee, and he was bothered with a lot of sweating.

His weight was 111 kilograms (17 stone 7), BMI 35 and his waist was 116 centimetres (45.6 inches). (From a health point of view, this measurement should have been less than 94 centimetres (37 inches).) Blood pressure was normal, 120/80 mm Hg. Blood tests showed excessive values of C-peptide, uric acid, homocysteine and an unfavourable profile of fats (lipids) in the blood (see pages 280, 285 and 283). Tomas had an increased risk of heart attack and good reason to be concerned.

He was informed of the relationships between food, blood sugar and insulin. I advised him to drastically reduce his consumption of bread, potatoes and foods containing sugar. He was also willing to cut down on coffee and Diet Coke. I also asked him to look at his work situation and to reduce the level of stress as much as possible. For many people stress can really slow down weight loss. Stress leads to increased cortisol production, and cortisol makes blood sugar and the insulin levels increase.

Blood test results before and after diet change.

Blood test	Before	After 3 months	Reference range
C-peptide (pmol/L)	1148	791	< 700
Total cholesterol (mmol/L)	6.3	5.2	2.9–6.1
HDL cholesterol (mmol/L)	0.7	0.7	0.8–2.1
LDL cholesterol (mmol/L)	4.5	3.9	1.2–4.3
Triglycerides (mmol/L)	2.47	1.62	< 1.7
Uric acid (µmol/L)	539	449	230–480
Homocysteine (µmol/L)	22.8	15.8	5–15

Tomas lost 3 kilograms (6.6 pounds) the first week and was very pleased. We agreed that he would reduce his carbohydrate consumption further. He ate a type of yogurt containing muesli, nuts, fruit, berries and sugar for breakfast. I recommended an omelette instead, because this yogurt contains a lot of carbohydrates. He had decided to start exercise again and had exchanged Diet Coke for mineral water. After three months, his blood tests were considerably improved and the risk of cardiovascular disease reduced. Four months after he had started on the diet, he weighed 20 kilograms (3 stone 2) less. He trained regularly, felt very good and sweated less. All in all, Tomas reduced his weight to 83 kilograms (13 stone 1), a total loss of 28 kilograms (4 stone 6).

Unfavourable blood fats profile

When there is more glucose than necessary for the production of energy, the liver converts the surplus to, among other things, triglycerides (fat) and cholesterol, which are transported out into the body. This leads to the concentration of triglycerides and cholesterol increasing in the blood. A high level of triglycerides and LDL cholesterol and a low level of HDL cholesterol is considered detrimental with regard to cardiovascular disease. Many studies have shown that the concentration of triglycerides is reduced with the consumption of few carbohydrates, and several studies have also shown that the cholesterol levels are greatly improved on a low carb diet. From experience, it takes a while before the concentration of HDL cholesterol increases.

Excessive level of homocysteine

The amino acid homocysteine is a recognised contributor to cardiovascular disease, and the level in the blood is normally reduced with the consumption of one, or sometimes three, key B vitamins (folate, B6 and B12). Consumption of B vitamins will, however, not necessarily reduce the risk for cardiovascular disease because the cause can be something else. Tomas didn't take B vitamin supplements, but as you see from the former table, the level of homocysteine was significantly reduced when he ate low carbohydrate food.

Consequences of being overweight and obesity

Next to smoking, obesity and obesity-related diseases are the most important indirect causes of premature death. The underlying reason, as a rule, is an excessive consumption of high carbohydrate food. There are clear connections between obesity and diseases such as cardiovascular disease, cancer, repetitive strain injuries, biliary disorders, sleep apnoea, mental disorders, diabetes and other hormonal disorders. It is not the obesity in itself, but the hormonal and biochemical changes which contribute to obesity, that cause most problems. The risk of contracting these secondary diseases increases with an increasing degree of obesity. Studies have shown that people who are already overweight in adolescence (14–19 years of age), have a higher risk of death from a range of diseases in adulthood. In other words, there is every reason to avoid being overweight or obese and to lose weight if you are in the danger zone.

Surveys show that people with obesity have a poorer quality of life than people of normal weight. In many cases, they also have a lower quality of life than other chronically ill patient groups. People who are overweight or obese often feel that they are victims of prejudice. Many people believe them to be lazy and inactive and that they eat cakes, ice cream and buns all day long. Although this of course applies to some, it is my experience that most people eat so-called good diets.

It is difficult to calculate how much obesity costs a society, but the direct and indirect costs are considerable.

High blood pressure

What is high blood pressure?

High blood pressure means that the pressure in the body's blood vessels is higher than what is defined as normal. Blood pressure is indicated by two numbers separated by a forward slash. The upper pressure (systolic pressure) is the pressure in the blood vessels when the heart contracts. The lower pressure (diastolic pressure) is the pressure in the blood vessels when the heart relaxes and fills with blood. High blood pressure usually gives no symptoms, but with very high pressure you can get a headache and become dizzy.

High blood pressure is very common. Many take blood pressure medication and any number of people have it without knowing it. It is estimated that more than 90 percent of everyone who is examined for high blood pressure has no reliable, provable cause. More often than not, high blood pressure is a result of several factors, where diet, exercise, being overweight and being stressed have the greatest significance. If you have an inherited tendency, it often means that there is nothing wrong with your genes but, rather, how they are expressed. This is, again, independent of our lifestyle. A normal blood pressure is 120/80 mm Hg or even a little lower. In our modern society, blood pressure often increases with age, but it doesn't among so-called primitive people who have a natural lifestyle. The figure on the next page shows systolic blood pressure with increasing age among men and women (in Norway).

High blood pressure is not regarded as a disease but as a risk factor that can contribute to a variety of diseases. The risk of having a stroke or developing heart disease, for instance, increases with increasing blood pressure. People who have had high blood pressure for many years often get a thickening of the wall in the left ventricle. This is a sign that the heart is being too heavily taxed.

Traditional medical treatment of high blood pressure

The boundaries for when high blood pressure should be treated are constantly being discussed in medical circles. If your blood pressure is very high, you will be advised to start treatment with medication quickly. If you have moderately high blood pressure, the doctor will undertake an overall assessment based on age and gender and other risk factors, such as hereditary factors, bodyweight, cholesterol levels, whether or not you smoke, exercise habits and diabetes. The doctor will often give lifestyle advice such as slimming (dieting), stopping smoking and getting more exercise, before you potentially begin with medication. Traditionally, a low calorie diet is recommended, with lots of carbohydrates and little fat for patients who need to lose weight.

Ivar wanted to stop using medicine for high blood pressure

Ivar was 62 years of age when he came for a consultation because he needed help reducing his weight. He also had a strong wish to stop using the medication he was taking for high blood pressure. There were many overweight people in Ivar's family. His sister also had high blood pressure.

Rising systolic blood pressure with increasing age among men and women in Norway.

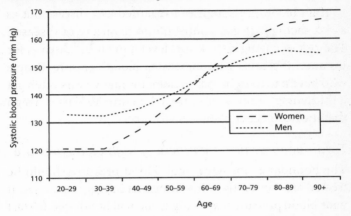

Source: The Norwegian Institute of Public Health, www.fhi.no

When he was in his 20s, he was very active in athletics, weighed 72 kilograms (11 stone 5) and had a BMI of 23. Gradually, his weight started to increase, and in his 50s, snoring became his main problem. It was so bad that he had to have his own bedroom so as not to wake up his wife. He had three laser treatments of his palate which provided a little improvement, but he still couldn't share a bed with his spouse. When he was 59, his wife discovered by chance that he had long pauses in his breathing at night, combined with the snoring. He got in touch with a private sleep laboratory to have this examined more closely. It was established that there were many, long pauses in his breathing, and he started with a C-PAP mask to aid his breathing. This worked well and also led to the snoring disappearing. He slept better and felt more rested when he woke. Ivar was able to share a bed with his wife again, even though the breathing apparatus made a little noise.

Ivar ate typical European food – high carb, low fat. On the weekends, he ate a little chocolate or a small piece of cake. He didn't exercise but, as a rule, went for a hike every weekend. He was concerned for his health because he was overweight and had to use high blood pressure medication. This meant that he had to stop donating blood, which he regretted.

When he came to me, he weighed 105 kilograms (16 stone 7). His BMI was 34. His blood pressure was 140/90 mm Hg when he was using the blood pressure medication. The blood tests showed that he had insulin resistance with excessive levels of C-peptide and insulin (see page 280).

Ivar wanted a quick weight loss and started, therefore, with a low calorie, low carb diet of the type VLCD (see page 232). He returned after four weeks and reported that the diet had been easy to follow. He hadn't been bothered by hunger and thought the products tasted fine. His weight had decreased by all of 9.9 kilograms (1 stone 8), of which 7.5 kilograms (16.5 pounds) was fat and 2.4 kilograms (5.3 pounds) was water. He noticed that he had markedly less fluid in his face and fingers. He said that he had stopped with the blood pressure medication on his own initiative a week before the check-up to see what happened. We were both excited when I measured his blood pressure, and to our great joy, it was now 120/80 mm Hg. He then replaced one powder meal with a meal consisting of meat or fish and vegetables and then came for a check-up after another five weeks. At that time, he had lost another 6.2 kilograms (nearly a stone), of which 5.6 kilograms (about 12 pounds) was fat and the rest water. In total, he had reduced his weight by 16.1 kilograms (2 stone 7) in nine weeks. Ivar replaced another powder meal with low carbohydrate food, and at the following check-up after six weeks, he had gone down four more kilograms (8.8 pounds). His blood pressure was now 110/70 mm Hg without the blood pressure medication.

Ivar was very pleased with his weight loss of 20 kilograms (3 stone 2) and a pill-free daily routine. His wife was happy because he did fine without the C-PAP mask at night. His goal was to lose another five kilograms (11 pounds) in order to reach his match weight of 80 kilograms (12 stone 8). He wanted to do this on his own over a period.

Blood test results before and after diet change.

Blood test	Before	After 3 months	Reference range
Blood sugar (mmol/L)	5.0	4.0	4–6
Long term blood sugar (%)	5.6	5.3	< 6.1
C-peptide (pmol/L)	1331	869	< 700
Insulin (pmol/L)	235	33	< 120

Sleep apnoea
– transient breathing pauses

About 4 percent of all men and 2 percent of all women aged 30–79 are affected by sleep apnoea. If the muscles in the airways relax too much at night, it can lead to the airways becoming too narrow. Snoring is often the result. If the airways are blocked entirely, breathing stops. This pause in breathing is called apnoea and can last between ten seconds and one minute. In the worst case, the pause can occur several hundred times each night. With repeated pauses, sleep is greatly disturbed, and you don't get the rest you need. The reduced oxygen level in the body results in the heart being forced to work harder, and both blood pressure and the level of stress hormones increase.

Several studies show that sleep apnoea often occurs simultaneously with high blood pressure, cardiovascular disease, diabetes and depression. C-PAP is the preferred treatment for severe or moderately severe sleep apnoea. The treatment consists of sleeping with a mask or nose pad that via a hose and a compressor creates a slight pressure. This keeps the upper airways open. The treatment is effective, and one experiences a rapid improvement in sleep quality and quality of life. Many overweight people have sleep apnoea, and as you can see by Ivar's history, weight loss can be effective both for doing away with sleep apnoea and for reducing blood pressure. It's worth noting that his blood pressure was normalised long before Ivar was cured of sleep apnoea.

Sugar, insulin and high blood pressure

The interior of the blood vessels produces a substance called nitrogen oxide (NO), which makes the blood vessels relax. Nitrogen oxide can therefore increase the flow of blood in the blood vessels and reduce the blood pressure. Insulin stimulates the release of NO.

With insulin resistance, the insulin doesn't work as it should (read more about insulin resistance on page 291), resulting in the blood vessels constricting and the blood pressure increasing.

A sufficient level of magnesium is also important for keeping blood pressure at a normal level. Magnesium plays a role in relaxing the muscels in the blood vessels. If you have too little magnesium in your body, it can result in your blood vessels constricting. This contributes to blood pressure increase. If you eat a lot of carbohydrates, you may have a magnesium deficiency (see page 215).

A lot of insulin causes the kidneys to excrete less salt, and as a result unnecessarily large amounts of salt and fluid accumulate in the body. This also contributes to blood pressure increasing. Insulin also causes inflammation reactions in the vessels, increased cell growth and consequently constricted blood vessels, which can lead to heart attack. The longer the blood pressure has been high, the more difficult it is to get it back to normal. This is due to the changes that have developed in the blood vessel walls.

Elise had high blood pressure and wanted to lose weight

Elise was 39 years old when she came for a consultation because she needed help to reduce her weight. She also had a strong desire to stop using the two blood pressure medications she was using. Elise's father had a lot of fat on his stomach, and many in her family had heart disease. She herself had had pre-eclampsia in her first pregnancy. Elise had steadily put on weight since her first pregnancy and, in the last few years she had a great craving for sweets. She was constantly tired, and her memory had become conspicuously poor. Her weight was 105 kilograms (16 stone 7) and her BMI was 38. Her blood pressure, while using two types of medication, was 140/85 mm Hg. Her waist measured 108 centimetres (42.5 inches), but it should have been under 88 centimetres (34.6 inches) and preferably under 80 centimetres (31.5 inches).

I explained to Elise how the body's blood sugar control worked, and I suspected that her problems were due to the fact that she ate more carbohydrates than she tolerated. She herself wished to try a low calorie/low carb VLCD diet (see page 232), which she had read about on the Internet. I supported her in this choice but explained that she must first gradually reduce the consumption of carbohydrates in her daily diet, and that I had to evaluate the blood test results before we started with the powder diet.

The blood tests showed that C-peptide was in the boundary area, the values for SHBG and vitamin D were too low, and the uric acid level was too high (see page 280, 288, 289 and 285). Too much insulin hampers the production of SHBG in the liver, and this leads to an increased amount of free testosterone in the blood. So even though Elise's insulin production wasn't particularly high, it was enough to result in hormone problems. Since it was winter, I recommended a supplement of vitamin D in the form of tablets.

Elise returned after two weeks and had reduced her weight by 2.5 kilograms (5.5 pounds) just by eating fewer carbohydrates. She was given information about low carb/low calorie powder diet she was going to use, and she was ready to get started. Four weeks on VLCD resulted in a weight loss of 11 kilograms (1 stone 10), of which 8 kilograms (1 stone 4) was fat and 3 kilograms (6.6 pounds) was water. It was a large weight loss in such a short time, but she had felt well and hadn't been hungry. Her blood pressure had dropped to 122/86 mm Hg. I asked her to replace one of the powder meals with meat or fish and vegetables that grow above ground. In addition, she was to take an extra salt supplement based on changes in her blood test results.

After another six weeks, she had lost another five kilograms (11 pounds), a total weight loss of 18 kilograms (2 stone 12) in two months. Her blood tests were normalised, and her blood pressure was 120/80 mm Hg, but she had measured lower values at home. We agreed that she was to stop using one of her medications and check her blood pressure carefully. If it was still normal, she could cut the other medication by half and perhaps quit it entirely. She did as I said and gets along now without blood pressure medication. After a gradual transition to an ordinary low carb diet, Elise continued losing weight on her own, without the need for any more consultations.

Elise had previously reduced her weight by 20 kilograms (3 stone 2) on a low fat, high carb diet, without being able to discontinue her blood pressure medicines. On a low carb diet, however, she was able to stop using the medications because the quantity of insulin in her body was reduced. A large amount of insulin is, as mentioned, often the reason for high blood pressure because it leads to a constriction of the blood vessels and accumulation of fluid in the body.

Blood test results before and after diet change.

Blood test	Before	After 3 months	Reference range
C-peptide (pmol/L)	677	512	< 700
SHBG (nmol/L)	16	36	23–100
Vitamin D_3 (nmol/L)	46	74	50 – 150

Pre-eclampsia

Women with pre-eclampsia have higher insulin values than healthy women. High insulin concentrations among healthy women early in pregnancy often means that they put on more weight during the pregnancy and have a higher weight after giving birth.

In a large study where women with severe pre-eclampsia were compared with women with uncomplicated pregnancies, the risk for high blood pressure tripled. Increased mortality from cardiovascular disease has also been reported among women who previously had pre-eclampsia. Obesity and metabolic syndrome (see page 293) are associated with the increased occurrence of pregnancy complications and birth defects: there is an increased risk of spontaneous abortion in the first three months of pregnancy. Later in the pregnancy, the risk of gestational diabetes, high blood pressure, pre-eclampsia and foetal death increases.

Diabetes

What is diabetes?

Diabetes mellitus, as it is actually called, means "sweet urine", a characteristic feature that doctors found among people with diabetes. In past times, doctors would taste a patient's urine to determine whether there was too much sugar in the urine! If the blood sugar becomes too high, the kidneys excrete sugar into the urine; this is a reaction imposed by evolution because too much sugar is dangerous for the body. Today diabetes mellitus is often just called "diabetes" or the "sugar disease". Diabetes is divided into four main groups, as you can see below.

The four groups of diabetes.

Group	Distinctive features of the disease
Type 1 diabetes	Reduced or no insulin production
Type 2 diabetes	Insulin resistance and decreased insulin response
Other types of diabetes	Genetic defects, various diseases in the pancreas
Gestational diabetes	Insulin resistance

In order to diagnose diabetes, the doctor must conduct a fasting test for sugar (glucose) in the blood or a glucose tolerance test where the blood sugar is measured two hours after the consumption of 75 grams of glucose. The doctor looks for how the body handles this load. The table on the next page shows the values which are defined as diabetes and decreased sugar tolerance.

Values which show diabetes and decreased sugar tolerance.

Diabetes	
Fasting glucose	7.0 mmol/L or higher
And/or value 2 hours after consumption of 75 grams of glucose	11.1 mmol/L or higher
And/or randomly taken glucose test in combination with symptoms	11.1 mmol/L or higher
Decreased sugar tolerance	
Fasting glucose	Less than 7.0 mmol/L
And value 2 hours after consumption of 75 grams of glucose	7.8 mmol/L or more, but less than 11.1 mmol/L

Source: Norwegian Directorate of Health 2009, IS-1674: Diabetes. Forebygging, diagnostikk og behandling ("Diabetes. Prevention, diagnosis and treatment").

Decreased sugar tolerance indicates that you are on your way to diabetes (pre-diabetes). Studies show that there are just as many people who have pre-diabetes as have diabetes.

The number of diabetics is rising

Diabetes is increasing all over the world; this applies to both type 1 and type 2. The World Health Organization (WHO) has published these figures for the number of cases of diabetes:

1985: 30 million
1995: 135 million
2000: 171 million
2030: 366 million (estimate)

Type 1 diabetes

Type 1 diabetes often starts in childhood and adolescence and was previously called insulin-dependent diabetes or juvenile diabetes. The disease develops because varying numbers of the insulin-producing cells in the pancreas have been destroyed by the body's own immune system, so that the pancreas cannot produce sufficient insulin. The reason that the cells are destroyed has not been definitively explained, but there are many hypotheses. Some studies indicate that the combination of peptides (chains of amino acids) from undigested proteins and leakage in the intestine (which results in these peptides being taken up in the blood) can lead to the body attacking and destroying the pancreas with its own immune apparatus. Other studies indicate that a deficiency of vitamin D in infancy appears to increase the risk of developing the disease. Viral infections during foetal (fetal) life or in early childhood are also regarded as a possible explanation. The British doctor Thomas Latimore Cleave showed that type 1 diabetes rarely occurs among hunter gatherers, but that the disease pops up 20–30 years after they begin using sugar and flour in their diet.

Symptoms of type 1 diabetes

The most common symptoms of type 1 diabetes are frequent urination, thirst, laxity, weight loss, frequent urinary tract infections and itchiness in the crotch. The symptoms often appear more suddenly and are more pronounced than with type 2 diabetes. If you don't get help from a doctor in time, you can get symptoms such as breathing difficulty, stomach pains, nausea and retching. Worst case, a patient might lose consciousness due to the combination of high blood sugar from lack of insulin and the acidification of the blood (diabetic ketoacidosis). In such instances, it is important to receive insulin immediately in order to normalise the blood sugar, along with fluids and minerals (salts).

Traditional medical treatment of type 1 diabetes

The traditional medical treatment for type 1 diabetes is insulin. Eating a diet of carbohydrates from fibre-rich foods with little fat is also recommended.

Kirsten had type 1 diabetes for 15 years and put on 30 kilograms (4 stone 10)

Kirsten came down with type 1 diabetes when she was 22 years old. She had two healthy children, and the pregnancies had gone well under strict medical monitoring. She weighed 70 kilograms (11 stone) before she got diabetes, but in the course of the 15 years she had used insulin, her weight had increased by 30 kilograms (4 stone 10). She used long-acting and fast-acting insulin, but despite long experience she was still plagued with low blood sugar (trembling, unease, perspiration). Her blood sugar was often down to 2.5 mmol/L, and then she felt very unwell and had a tendency to eat too many sweets, so that her blood sugar was suddenly 10 mmol/L. She was, otherwise, a very controlled person, was very careful with what she ate and tried to keep her blood sugar as normal as possible. Kirsten ate as she had learnt from the Norwegian Diabetes Association, and her diet consisted of slices of bread for breakfast and lunch, a dinner with vegetables and potatoes, rice or pasta and slices of bread for her evening meal. She ate two pieces of fruit a day.

The week before she came to me, she had reduced her consumption of carbohydrates, which had led to her needing only half as much fast-acting insulin. I carefully explained to her the connection between carbohydrates, blood sugar and the need for insulin. I asked her to read the book written by the American doctor Richard Bernstein *(The Diabetes Solution)*, because it explains this interaction so well. I pointed out how important it was that the amount of insulin be reduced so that she would be able to lose the weight. The goal before the next check-up was to maintain her blood sugar within the normal range and further reduce her intake of carbohydrates. I told her that natural fat is a perfect food source for diabetics because it does not affect the blood sugar at all. She wanted, therefore, to try to eat more fat, even though it conflicted with everything she had learnt. She was fond of butter, cream, sour cream, cheese, avocado and oily fish, so she figured that it would go well. I encouraged her to keep a diary of what she ate and which insulin doses she took, and to write down all her blood sugar measurements so that we had a good basis for discussion next time.

When she returned after four weeks, we reviewed the blood test results first. Considering the fact that she had type 1 diabetes and used insulin, her long-term blood sugar was fine. She did, however, have some low blood sugar values in the period before she took the samples, which indicate that she must also have had some high levels in order to get a long-term blood sugar of 7.1 percent. A long-term blood sugar of 7 percent corresponds to an average blood sugar of 8.3 mmol/L (see page 279). The blood samples were taken in the spring, and her level of vitamin D was too low. I recommended a supplement and sunbathing in the summer. Her selenium level was also relatively low, and we agreed that she should take a multivitamin tablet and two Brazil nuts daily (see page 288).

In the course of the past few weeks, she had further reduced her consumption of carbohydrates, and so had again halved her doses of fast-acting insulin. She had also reduced her long-acting insulin by four units. Her blood sugar had been between 5 and 6 mmol/L, and she had reduced her weight by 6 kilograms (13 pounds) in six weeks. She felt much fitter but needed a little inspiration for cooking, so I recommended a couple of cookbooks with low carb food. After another four weeks, she had taken off another 3 kilograms (6.5 pounds) and felt that this was very motivating. She had been to her regular doctor in the meantime, who was positive to the plan once she saw the fine results. Kirsten had found the key to reducing her weight and keeping her blood sugar stable. Further monitoring of her diabetes is taking place under the care of her regular doctor.

Experiences with low carb diet and insulin doses

The amount of insulin people with type 1 diabetes need is dependent on how many carbohydrates they eat and how much insulin the pancreas continues to be able to produce. My experience and that of others shows that many can cut the amount of insulin they must inject by between 50 and 80 percent when they change to a low carb diet. There are also examples of people with type 1 diabetes having managed completely without insulin for many years. This assumes, of course, that they have a certain production of insulin themselves. If you have type 1 diabetes and wish to try a low carb diet, it is extremely important that you work together with a physician.

Insulin and weight gain

Good blood sugar control for patients with diabetes is extremely important because it prevents or reduces deferred complications such as eye, kidney and nerve damage. A high carbohydrate consumption and insulin level can, however, lead to insulin resistance. This leads to a need for larger doses of insulin to keep the blood sugar down. Insulin-related weight gain is explained by among other things, its anabolic (building-up) and appetite-increasing effect.

Calculating carbohydrates and dosage of insulin

Estimating how many carbohydrates there are in a meal and determining an insulin dose accordingly is not easy. If you're really good at it, you can calculate the carbohydrate amount at 150 grams with a margin of error of 20 percent. Which amounts to a margin of error of 30 grams of carbohydrates. Let's say that you think it's 150 grams, but that in reality it's 180 grams. If you are a slim person with type 1 diabetes and do not produce insulin, 1 gram of carbohydrates will increase your blood sugar by nearly 0.3 mmol/L. Thirty grams, then, will increase your blood sugar by 9 mmol/L (0.3 x 30). If at the outset you had a normal blood sugar level of 5 mmol/L, ate 180 grams of carbohydrates and determined an insulin dose for 150 grams of carbohydrates, your blood sugar would have increased from 5 to approximately 14 mmol/L (5 + 9). If on the other hand you thought that you ate more carbohydrates than you actually did, your blood sugar would have dipped, and you probably would have developed hypoglycaemia (trembling, unease, perspiration) and would have to eat sugary food to prevent it from really going downhill. Both situations result in you having problems with blood sugar the rest of the day. If you calculate 20 percent wrong on average, sometimes you will calculate 10 percent wrong and other times 30 percent. So, the problem here is that the delivery of large amounts of carbohydrates results in large fluctuations in blood sugar.

Let's say that you ate a salad instead and calculated that there were 12 grams of carbohydrates in the salad. Let's say that you calculated a full 30 percent wrong. Then you would have made a calculation error that constituted only of 4 grams of carbohydrates. That results in an increase or a decrease in the blood sugar of just 1.2 mmol/L (0.3 x 4). Meaning that it is much easier to determine a dose of insulin and have stable blood sugar with a low consumption of carbohydrates. With radical changes in diet, I recommend monitoring by a physician.

Type 2 diabetes

Type 2 diabetes was previously seen only among the elderly, and the disease was most common among women. There is still a strong increase with increasing age, but the youngest people getting the disease now are under 20 years old. Today more men in all age groups are stricken, which fits with the fact that the "obesity epidemic" has lasted longer and is somewhat more pronounced among men than among women. An exception is women from Pakistan and India, because they are more predisposed than men. The main cause of this disease is a lifestyle dominated by incorrect diet, lack of exercise and lots of stress. The disease expresses itself in insulin resistance – the cells that have receptors for insulin become less sensitive. The pancreas tries to counteract this by secreting more insulin, which can "tire" the cells, so that the pancreas becomes poorer at sending insulin out to the blood. Consequently, the problem becomes even more dangerous, and so many elderly people with type 2 diabetes become insulin users, which they must continue as long as they continue to burden the body with too much carbohydrates.

Symptoms of type 2 diabetes

The symptoms of type 2 diabetes can be faint in the beginning, so that patients often go a long time with the disease without being aware that they have it. On average, a patient develops the precursor to diabetes 10–15 years before the disease breaks out in earnest. Often type 2 diabetes is first discovered when complications and related diseases appear – for example, a heart attack. If the blood sugar becomes sufficiently high, patients develop sugar in the urine and symptoms such as frequent urination, thirst, fatigue, itching in the crotch, repeated urinary tract infections and weight loss.

Traditional medical treatment of type 2 diabetes

Foods with lots of carbohydrates from fibre-rich foods and reduced fat are generally recommended. Weight reduction with low calorie, high carb diets, medications or surgery are recommended in the event of patients being overweight and obese. Physical activity and stopping smoking are advised. If the goal of a long-term blood sugar level below 7 percent is not reached in the course of three months, patients are recommended to start taking medication. If this still doesn't work, insulin injections are then recommended.

Astrid didn't know she had diabetes

Astrid was 43 years old when she consulted me because she wanted to lose weight. She had been plump as long as she could remember, and childhood photos showed that she had been that way since she was two years old. When she became pregnant, she gained a lot of weight. She didn't get rid of all the weight before the next pregnancy. There were many obese people in the family, on both her mother and her father's side. No one in the family had diabetes, but many had suffered heart attacks in their 50s and 60s. Astrid had, for a long time, felt unusually tired, her stomach was always bloated, and her bowel movements alternated between being loose and hard. She had a lot of fluid in her body and was plagued with painful, stiff fingers. At times she had large outbreaks of eczema and had gone through several rounds of cortisone treatment. At these times she had noticed that she put on a little extra weight. When I first met her, she was on sick leave.

Astrid weighed 133 kilograms (20 stone 13), she had a BMI of 47, and her blood pressure was too high at 160/90 mm Hg. We agreed that she would reduce her consumption of carbohydrates dramatically down to about 20 grams per day after one week (ketogenic diet, see page 229). She wondered if she should start exercising, and I advised her to walk three times a week at a tempo that felt comfortable. She could intensify her training after she had lost 10–20 kilograms (20 to 40 pounds). She thought that was a good plan, because exercising with her large body was difficult.

After four weeks, she returned and reported that she had started right on the ketogenic diet the day after she had been to see me. She didn't have any problems with it and felt better from the first day. To her great surprise the eczema disappeared in the course of the first week. For breakfast she had eaten avocado, cottage cheese and shrimp. Lunch consisted often of a salad with tuna or egg, and for dinner she ate meat or fish and plenty of vegetables. If she was hungry in the evening, she had a little cottage cheese, cheese or eggs in one or another form. Her weight was reduced by 7 kilograms (1 stone 1) during these four weeks.

We went through the blood tests that she had taken after she had been to see me. They showed that she had far too high levels of sugar, C-peptide, uric acid and Micro-CRP, and insufficient levels of vitamin D and SHBG. Astrid wasn't so surprised that I had confirmed diabetes. She had indeed thought that she was in the risk group since she was so overweight. I urged her to continue with the diet and explained that her blood sugar was probably fine after four weeks on ketogenic diet. In addition, I recommended some dietary supplements, to improve her vitamin and anti-oxidant values. I gave her a recipe for low carb bread, to give her a little more variety in her diet. During the next five weeks she lost four more kilograms (9 pounds) she felt very well and decided that she would start exercising at a fitness centre. Her blood pressure had normalised.

After five months, she was 25 kilograms (3 stone 13) lighter, and the blood test results were much better. It takes a little time for all the tests to normalise when the weight is so great. The concentration of vitamin D was still too low, and since it was early spring, I advised her to double her dose until the summer. The level of uric acid and Micro-

CRP was still too high, but that is consistent with her insulin still being above the normal level.

On this diet, Astrid no longer had diabetes, which motivated her to continue eating this way. She had understood how to lose weight and avoid diabetes, and now she wanted to try and manage on her own.

Blood test results before and after diet change.

Blood test	Before	After 5 months	Reference range
Blood sugar (mmol/L)	11.0	5.9	4–6
Long-term blood sugar (%)	8.4	5.3	< 6.1
C-peptide (pmol/L)	1728	994	< 700
SHBG (nmol/L)	18	36	23–100
Micro-CRP (mg/L)	14	9	<5
Uric acid (µmol/L)	371	366	155–350
Vitamin D_3 (nmol/L)	34	47	50–150

Sugar, insulin and type 2 diabetes

Type 2 diabetes develops from having too many carbohydrates in the diet. We are not made for eating large quantities of carbohydrates, and they quite simply have overwhelmed the body's natural ability to handle sugar. Type 2 diabetes is the final stage of insulin resistance.

People with type 2 diabetes may have high, normal or low insulin production. Most of them have a high insulin level and put on a lot of weight on a typical modern diet, because insulin stimulates the body to store fat, but inhibits it from burning fat. With insulin injections, insulin production may be normal, because the pancreas doesn't need to work as hard to produce insulin when it is delivered externally. Stoping insulin injections will often cause the pancreas to increase production. This happens because the body is very insulin resistant, and a lot of insulin is required to keep the blood sugar under control. With a low carb diet and weight loss, however, the body will become more sensitive to the effect of insulin. The blood sugar will normalise provided that the body itself produces sufficient insulin. About 20 percent of those who get diabetes at an adult age are slim. Their pancreas doesn't produce very much insulin. They may have insulin resistance aren't able to compensate by producing enough insulin. This results in them getting diabetes more quickly than people who produce large quantities of insulin. These people often manage fine on a low carb diet if they still produce sufficient insulin.

Good blood sugar control is important for diabetics. It prevents or reduces complications such as eye, kidney and nerve damage. Treatment with insulin is, however, not unproblematic, because a lot of insulin often leads to weight gain. Weight gain also plays a role in increased insulin resistance and increased risk of cardiovascular disease.

Normal and decreased insulin response

Before I tell you what is meant by decreased insulin response, I have to say a little about how the production of insulin occurs in a person who doesn't have diabetes. In a fasting person without diabetes, the pancreas continuously releases a little insulin, so that the insulin level is at a stable, low level. This base line level of insulin prevents the liver from transforming amino acids from the body's proteins (from, for example, muscles) into glucose so that the blood sugar rises. A healthy, slim person without diabetes usually has a blood sugar level that stays within narrow boundaries, fluctuating relatively little.

**Phase 1 and Phase 2 insulin response
in a person who does not have diabetes.**

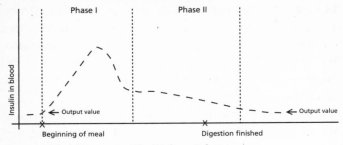

Source: Richard Bernstein: The Diabetes Solution

When you eat a breakfast consisting of one slice of bread with egg and one slice of bread with preserves, the following happens: The sugar that comes from the bread and the preserves enters the blood stream quickly, and the pancreas responds by releasing insulin which it has stored. This rapid release of stored insulin is called insulin reaction phase 1 (see the figure above). When the pancreas uses its stored insulin, it starts to produce more, and when this insulin is released, it's called Phase 2 insulin response. The newly-produced insulin is secreted much more slowly than that which is stored. So this insulin can deal with the sugar that is slowly being produced from proteins in the meal. Some of the sugar is converted to glycogen and is stored in the muscles and the liver for later use. If there is still abundant sugar in the blood, it is converted to fat. If it is a long time to the next meal, and the blood sugar starts to fall, the glycogen will be converted to glucose again to raise the blood sugar level.

If you have a depressed insulin response, the pancreas has little or no stored insulin that can be released rapidly into the blood when you eat carbohydrates. It's like this because the pancreas works hard around the clock to produce all the insulin that's required to have some effect on the insulin-resistant cells. Phase 2 insulin response can function okay, and the pancreas will slowly produce the amount of insulin that is necessary to lower blood sugar again. But then the blood sugar level could have been high for several hours, which is damaging to the body.

The figure on the next page shows that an overweight person produces two to three times as much insulin as a slim person. Overweight people with type 2 diabetes also produce a lot of insulin, but they lack the rapid Phase 1 insulin response. Thin people with type 2 diabetes produce less insulin than thin people without diabetes.

Insulin response in people with and without type 2 diabetes.

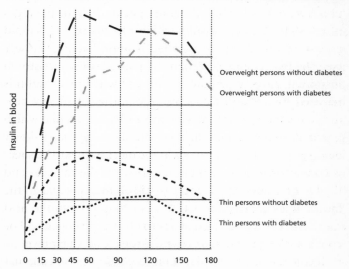

Source: Richard Bernstein: The Diabetes Solution

Many in Alf's family had diabetes

Alf was 47 years old and had felt tired for a long time. His vision had become weaker (he focused more poorly), he was often thirsty and constantly had to pass water. His sex life had begun to decline because of poor erectile function. Alf was eventually diagnosed with high blood sugar by his company doctor, and he was referred to a general practitioner (GP), urologist and ophthalmologist for further examination and treatment. He had an appointment with his GP's locum (substutute) a week later.

The blood test taken by the locum showed that Alf's fasting blood sugar was 3–4 times higher than normal, and sugar was confirmed in the urine. The locum called a university hospital and was advised to inform the patient that he had to stop eating sweets and start exercising. After two weeks, the patient came for a check-up with a new locum. His blood sugar was just as high, even though he hadn't eaten sweet foods and had exercised more than before. He was, therefore, referred to a university hospital but didn't hear anything from them. The doctor followed up on the referral and was informed that it had been forwarded to another university hospital, because that was where the patient belonged. About three months went by. The patient's blood sugar was between 15 and 17 mmol/L, and he felt awful all the time. Alf searched on the Internet to find help.

In Alf's family there are many who have type 2 diabetes. Several of them use insulin daily and a typical modern diet that includes cakes and sweets. Alf didn't want to end up like his relatives; he wanted to do what he could to get by without insulin. I asked Alf what he ate, and he said that he followed official guidelines for both diet and exercise. His meals consisted of wholemeal bread, orange juice, skimmed milk, fruit, rice, pasta, plenty of fish and vegetables. For snacks he ate dark chocolate and peanuts. He drank up to 1 litre of skimmed milk and played football twice a week. He had reduced his weight by approximately 10 kilograms (1 stone 8) the last year by improving his diet, and his BMI was 26, while his blood pressure was 160/95 mm Hg at the first consultation. He used no medicines. The blood tests that were taken a couple of days after the first consultation showed excessive levels of long-term blood sugar, C-peptide and triglycerides (see pages 279, 280 and 281).

I told Alf that he could get healthy if he removed most of the carbohydrates from his diet. The milk alone gave him nearly 50 grams of sugar a day, and he also got too much sugar from juice and fruit. He was getting plenty of starch from rice, pasta and bread, which was breaking down into sugar in his intestine. He was advised to eat mostly meat, fish, eggs, cheese, natural fats, nuts and vegetables. Furthermore, he should measure his blood sugar in the morning, evening and after all meals. He was also asked to keep a careful diary of everything he ate, his exercise activities and blood sugar measurements. I advised Alf to take the medication metformin initially to improve insulin resistance. I called him after a few days to hear how it was going. He reported that his blood sugar had fallen rapidly, and that he felt much better after having changed his diet. At a checkup one month later, his blood sugar was 8–9 mmol/L in the morning and 5–7 mmol/L in the evening. He had had an episode of hypoglycaemia (trembling, unease, perspiration) after taking a walk for exercise. His diet consisted mainly of fish, meat, cheese, crème fraîche, butter, olive oil, nuts, vegetables, berries, natural yogurt and some pulses.

I explained that his blood sugar was higher in the morning because he still had insulin resistance in his liver, which wasn't responding properly to the instructions from the insulin. In healthy people, insulin gives a signal to the liver not to pass sugar into the blood if there is already enough sugar there. With insulin resistance, this mechanism doesn't work properly, so the liver sends sugar to the blood, even though there is plenty of sugar already there. The episode with trembling, unease and perspiration reflected a rapid fall in his blood sugar level, even though it hadn't been lower than it normally was. If you have had high blood sugar for a long time, your body will interpret a rapid fall as having an abnormally low blood sugar level. The body tries to correct this by producing several hormones which promote an increase in the blood sugar once again. One of these hormones is adrenalin, which causes the symptoms mentioned. Eventually, as the blood sugar is normalised, the boundary for what the body perceives as abnormal is moved lower. A person with type 2 diabetes never gets dangerously low blood sugar unless he/she uses medication for lowering blood sugar (although this doesn't apply to metformin).

By changing his diet, Alf's vision and sexual potency gradually improved. A check of his blood pressure after three months showed that it had been reduced from 160/95 to 110/70 mm Hg; in other words, he had achieved a completely normal level without the use of blood pressure medication. He reduced his weight by 7 kilograms (1 stone 1), and his BMI was now 24. His long-term blood sugar was still a little too high after 3 months but was normal at a check-up after 18 months. His level of C-peptide and triglycerides was normalised after 3 months.

Alf was informed that he had to live on a low carbohydrate diet the rest of his life to stay healthy, and that he would develop diabetes again if he went back to his previous diet dominated by carbohydrates. Alf stated that he was shocked at politicians and at the official diabetes organisations, who recommend a diet which means that people remain dependent on insulin and medication.

Blood test results before and after diet change.

Blood test	Before	After 3 months	Reference range
Long-term blood sugar (%) (5.7 after 18 months)	10.6	6.5	< 6.1
C-peptide (pmol/L)	1215	516	< 700
Triglycerides (mmol/L)	2.61	1.01	< 1.7

High blood sugar and poor vision

When blood sugar levels are high, the concentration of sugar will also increase in the lens of the eye. This sugar attracts water, which results in the lens becoming rounder than usual, and it becomes more difficult to focus. The condition is reversed when the blood sugar is normalised, and the lens reverts to its normal shape.

High blood sugar and poor erections

High blood sugar inhibits the production and release of nitrogen oxide (NO), a molecule which normally promotes relaxation of the blood vessels. This leads to the penis not being filled with a sufficient quantity of blood upon sexual stimulation, and the erection is either poor or doesn't happen at all.

Pre-disposition for type 2 diabetes

Type 2 diabetes occurs far more often in some families than in others. If one of your parents has the disease, you have approximately a 40 percent risk of developing it yourself. If both your parents have type 2 diabetes, the risk is around 80 percent. It doesn't mean, however, that you automatically will get the disease, but the chance increases if your lifestyle is such that a hereditary pre-disposition is allowed to develop. The probability of getting the disease is far greater among those who have a lot of stomach fat, high blood pressure and an unfavourable profile of fats in the blood.

Are the official recommendations sound?

The Norwegian Diabetes Association writes that the cornerstones in the treatment of diabetes are motivation and knowledge, diet, physical activity and medication. They emphasise quitting smoking, losing weight and exercising. The object of the treatment of diabetes is two-fold. The short-term objective is daily well-being and freedom from symptoms. The long term objective is to prevent or delay the development of deferred complications.

The Norwegian Diabetes Association and the Norwegian National Council for Nutrition have a common understanding of what is the correct diet for diabetics. They recommend the same diet as for the rest of the population; 45–60 percentage of energy should come from carbohydrates, a maximum of 35 percentage from fat and 10–20 percentage from protein. Food should be spread between four to six meals per day. For those wishing to lose weight, reduced-energy diets are recommended, and the Norwegian National

Council for Nutrition has recently opened up to the idea that a diet with low carbohydrate content can be *also* used to lose weight for a period of up to one year. On the website of the Norwegian National Council for Nutrition, it states, however, that they do not primarily recommend such diets, but instead recommend reduced quantities of a regular varied diet in accordance with the general recommendations. The Norwegian National Council for Nutrition thinks, in fact, that such a diet has a much broader purpose than merely weight loss, namely to prevent chronic disease, cardiovascular disease, cancer and diabetes.

This council consists of ten members who primarily do research and teaching. The Council has limited experience in the treatment of patients with different diets. When you have read this book, you will see that all the patients I have written about came down with diseases and health problems even though, on the whole, they followed the advice of the authorities. The reason for this was invariably a high consumption of carbohydrates, leading to their insulin levels becoming too high. A lot of insulin leads to obesity and various diseases – which the Norwegian National Council for Nutrition thinks can be prevented with a high carb, low fat diet. I don't understand how anyone can continue to recommend a high carb diet to people who have become sick from eating too many carbohydrates! Nor do I understand, (since so many become sick from this diet) why this diet is recommended to the population in general. In my opinion, this advice leads to many people becoming overweight and sick. The dietary recommendations should at the very least be individualised.

In the brochure "Mat og type 2-diabetes" ("Food and Type 2 Diabetes") published by the Norwegian Diabetes Association, the reader learns that a diabetic should eat 1–3 slices of bread at each meal, at least 2 pieces of fruit each day, and for dinner 2–3 small potatoes, because they contain few calories and are very filling. They claim that this amount doesn't have any large effect on the blood sugar. At the back of the booklet, there is a recipe for carrot cake that contains 180 grams of flour and 120 grams of brown sugar. We are told that it isn't necessary to quit eating desserts and coffee treats even though we have diabetes.

Wholemeal bread is, of course, a better alternative than bread, but eating several slices usually results in a powerful blood sugar increase for diabetics. If you have it, you have perhaps noticed that your blood sugar increases a lot when you eat grain products, regardless of the type of diabetes. This is because grain contains a great deal of starch that turns up in the blood as glucose. The same applies to potatoes. It is glucose that is being measured when you take a blood sugar test.

If you have type 2 diabetes and you follow the traditional, official dietary advice your blood sugar levels will, as a rule, steadily increase. You will then be advised to take a tablet to lower your blood sugar and, after a while, a second tablet as well. Finally, you may be required to use insulin, which doesn't necessarily lead to good blood sugar control and which has the unfortunate effect of increasing your weight.

Before we had tablets to reduce blood sugar, people with type 2 diabetes were advised to weigh the bread and potatoes and other high carb foods so that carbohydrate consumption was so low that the body could handle it without elevataing the blood sugar. It's too bad that this advice has been stopped, because it actually worked well. A diabetic has become sick from sugar, and if you significantly reduce the consumption of sugary and starchy foods, then in most cases you get rid of the entire problem.

Listen to your own body

One day I had an elderly woman in the office, and she said that she had developed type 2 diabetes. She was a veteran nurse and thought back to how they learnt to treat diabetes patients when she was a student. She started to weigh high carb food so that she consumed approximately 40–50 grams carbohydrates per day, and to her great joy her blood sugar was normal in the course of a few days. She actually came to me to confirm that she was doing everything correctly. I did, of course, and told her that she could well eat strawberries all summer, but that she had to remember to have plenty of cream on them. When she came back for a check-up, she said that she had found her old lecture notes from the diabetes doctor, and there it said exactly what I had said; that fat inhibits the increase of blood sugar levels, and that people with diabetes should eat berries instead of other fruit (less sugar) and use plenty of cream.

Another time, I had a consultation with a man who had just started taking insulin for his type 2 diabetes. He had been to a diabetes class and learnt how much insulin he had to inject for each slice of bread he ate. It worked fairly well, but he was still not satisfied with his fluctuating blood sugar levels. So he wondered if two slices of bread required so much insulin, how much is required then for no bread? He tested this on himself and found that if he ate an omelette with vegetables he didn't need insulin for the meal at all. He thought this was a fine discovery but was amazed that he had had to find it out for himself.

If you have diabetes, I suggest that you do some tests on

yourself. Measure your blood sugar, eat meat, vegetables and three potatoes and measure your blood sugar every half hour until it normalises. Another day you can do the same test without potatoes and record what happens then. If you use insulin, you can record how much more insulin you need when you eat a meal with three potatoes, compared with a meal without potatoes. Fruit is a double-edged sword, particularly for diabetics. It tastes good and contains some vitamins, minerals and anti-oxidants, but the disadvantage is that fruit contains a lot of sugar. By using the summary of carbohydrate content in foods on page 294, you can figure out how many carbohydrates you get per day on your regular diet.

Linda followed a so-called diabetes diet but was unable to control her blood sugar

Linda was 60 years old and had been a very active and a social person. Her day was filled with a full-time job and many different social activities. However, the past year, she had felt worn out. She had difficulty breathing, felt weak, and she often got cramps in her legs. In addition, her weight had increased considerably over the last few years. She felt that something was seriously wrong and eventually contacted her regular doctor, who confirmed diabetes. He recommended treatment with medication, but Linda didn't want to take more medication than she already did. Instead she wanted to investigate whether there was something else she could do to improve the situation.

Linda was very concerned about her diagnosis, because her father had died from a stroke at age 57, and her mother died from a heart attack at age 65. Her brother was slim, but he also had diabetes. She herself had albumin in her urine during two pregnancies, high blood pressure, a high choles-terol count and a little asthma. Linda used one medication for high blood pressure and one for high cholesterol, in addi-tion to drugs for her asthma. She trained at a fitness centre twice a week and liked walking.

By a coincidence, she was advised to seek help from me. At that time, she weighed 86.2 kilograms (13 stone 8) and had a BMI of 28.5. Her blood pressure was normal when she used the blood pressure medication (115/85 mm Hg). Blood tests showed that she had excessive levels of sugar, C-peptide, ALAT and ferritin (see pages 279, 280, 285 and 284).

Linda ate the food she had been recommended by the Norwegian Diabetes Association but still didn't have good control over her blood sugar. I told her that it was entirely possible to get rid of diabetes if she was willing to make radical changes in her diet, to which she was extremely pos-itive. I advised her to stop eating food containing starch such as bread, potatoes, rice and pasta, so that within the course of a couple of weeks her carbohydrate consumption would be only about 20 grams per day. Linda was happy when she heard that she could eat a lot of eggs, meat, fish and cheese, because this was food she loved. She had low levels of certain vitamins and minerals, so I recommended several dietary supplements. Her GP was informed.

Linda thrived on the new diet, and after five months her weight had been reduced by 12 kilograms (1 stone 13). Her GP had reduced the strength of her blood pressure medication twice, and her blood pressure was as good as before. She now takes the lowest dose but doesn't dare com-pletely stop taking the medicine that she has used for over 20 years. Linda is happy with the outcome. The bonus was that she lost weight without thinking about dieting. In addition, she's now bursting with energy and has enough for all her activities. After nine months, her blood tests were normal except for C-peptide, which had been reduced but was still too high.

Blood test results before and after diet change.

Blood test	Before	After 3 months	Reference range
Long-term blood sugar (%)	6.9	6.0	< 6.1
C-peptide (pmol/L)	1164	984	< 700
Ferritin (µg/L)	187	81	13–150
ALAT (U/L)	48	30	8–46

Sequelae (Secondary diseases) to diabetes

Sugar in large quantities damages the blood vessel walls, and because people with type 1 and type 2 diabetes have elevated blood sugar, they have an increased risk of a range of sequelae or deferred complications. The most serious are kidney disease, strokes, heart cramps, heart attacks, eye damage, nerve damage, reduced circulation in the legs, erectile dysfunction in men and reduced sensitivity in the genitals in women. In order to prevent such complications, it's important to have as normal blood sugar levels as possible.

Kidney disease

With diabetic kidney damage, the smallest blood vessels in the kidneys are damaged. The first sign of kidney damage is leakage of proteins into the urine – first in small quantities (microalbuminuria) and later in larger quantities (proteinuria). A urine test is required for identification of proteins in the urine. The kidney function itself begins to shut down when proteinuria is present.

Stroke

With strokes a part of the brain becomes damaged. It can be because a blood vessel has become constricted, so that blood doesn't get to parts of the brain, or because a blood vessel is bleeding so that the blood flows out in the brain. The symptoms can be paralysis, impaired speaking ability, vision problems, severe headache, lethargy or unconsciousness. In the event of a stroke, admission to hospital and treatment can counteract complications.

Angina pectoris (heart cramp) and heart attack

A common symptom is pain or pressure in the centre or to the left of the chest. The pain often radiates out into either the left arm, both arms and/or the back and jaw. Angina pectoris often starts with pain during strenuous activity, that can be both physical and psychological. Eventually less strain causes pain, and finally there is also pain when one is resting. The pain with a heart attack is about the same as with angina pectoris, but it doesn't diminish while resting and is often more severe.

Individuals often experience these symptoms in drastically different ways. Women often have less typical and more diffuse symptoms than men; they may feel ill, develop nausea, stomach or back pain and having difficulty in breathing. The pain diabetics feel is more sneaking and diffuse, probably because the nerves that go to the heart have been damaged. Usually the cause is constrictions and/or blood clots in one or more of the coronary arteries. If one of these blood vessels becomes constricted or so narrow that the heart muscle doesn't get enough blood, tissue in the area that that vessel supplies with blood, will die. This is called a heart attack.

Anyone with severe angina pectoris or a heart attack must immediately be admitted to hospital. If you have diabetes, you have an increased risk of angina pectoris and heart attack, because you have higher blood sugar than people without diabetes, even if you're using blood sugar-reducing medicines. Diabetics also have high blood pressure, unfavourable fat values in the blood and often suffer from being overweight.

Eye damage

Chronic, elevated, or frequently high, blood sugar levels can result in changes in the small blood vessels in the eyes. The most common eye complication is changes to the retina (diabetic retinopathy) with the growth of new blood vessels that bleed easily and small haemorrhages from old vessels. The most important thing for preventing such complications is to keep the blood sugar as stable as possible. Preventive blood pressure treatment appears to have a positive effect on limiting the development of retinopathy. Diabetics can have changes in the back of the eyeball (fundus) without having symptoms in their eyes. Small changes don't necessarily require treatment, but the earlier the changes are diagnosed, the easier it is for the ophthalmologist to monitor progress and provide treatment when it becomes necessary. If you have type 1 diabetes, you ought to go to an ophthalmologist within five years of being diagnosed and annually thereafter. If you have type 2 diabetes, it is recommended that you go to an ophthalmologist immediately after you have received your diagnosis.

Neuropathy (nerve damage) and reduced blood circulation in the legs

Both neuropathy and changes in the blood vessels in the legs contribute to foot problems in diabetics. Neuropathy affects all types of nerves, and the nerve damage results in impairment of both the sense of touch and the ability to sense temperature in the legs and the feet. Feet with nerve damage are more sensitive to pressure, resulting in in hard skin. Haemorrhages develop under the hard skin, and infections can arise in these accumulations of blood.

Reduced blood circulation is due to the blood vessels being constricted, and this leads, among other things, to a reduction in the tissue's ability to repair wounds. Neuropathy and reduced blood circulation can, in the worst cases, lead to amputation. Everyone who suffers from diabetes should have their feet examined and get instruction in foot care at least once a year.

Erectile dysfunction

Erectile dysfunction is defined as the "deficient ability to have and/or maintain an erection that is sufficient for satisfying sexual activity." An erection results from a complex interplay between nerve signals and response in the musculature in the penis. When the brain registers sexual stimuli, it will set in motion a natural chemical process. This results in increased blood flow to the erectile tissue in the penis so that it becomes stiff. Problems with the blood supply and/or the nervous system can therefore lead to erectile dysfunction. The cause of erectile dysfunction among men with diabetes can be neuropathy, poor blood supply to the penis due to narrow blood vessels or various medicines.

There are several forms of treatment today for erectile dysfunction. If medication is not effective, there are various mechanical devices which can be tried.

Mari used insulin, gained weight and developed angina pectoris

Mari sought me out when she was 48 years old, because she was distraught over not being able to control her blood sugar, despite the fact that she took many injections of insulin every day. In addition, she gained weight even though she didn't eat much. She had tried countless diets without any of them having helped. Her legs were like logs, her energy level was at rock bottom, and her stomach was always bloated. She said that her natural weight at 20 had been 47 kilograms (7 stone 6). She contracted gestational diabetes in her second pregnancy but was told that her blood sugar would normalise after the delivery. It didn't, however, and she was diagnosed with type 2 diabetes when she was 36 years old. She was asked to reduce her consumption of sweets, but her blood sugar still gradually increased. She was advised to take metformin, which can improve insulin sensitivity and inhibit the production of sugar in the liver. She tried this but was so plagued with stomach pains that she had to quit the medicine.

Five years after the diagnosis, her general condition became gradually poorer and finally she was admitted to hospital. Her blood test showed a sky-high blood sugar of 27 mmol/L, and treatment with insulin was begun. The insulin doses had to be increased constantly to keep her blood sugar down. To Mari's great despair, her weight increased in parallel with the increasing insulin doses. Eventually she got high blood pressure, low metabolism and had to have her gall bladder removed because of gall stones which constantly gave her pain spasms. She was also plagued with a lot of pain in her joints and muscles. One day she had severe chest pains and was again admitted to hospital, where she had a metal tube (stent) inserted in a blood vessel to the heart to keep it open. She now used eleven different medications for these various disorders, of which four were for high blood pressure. She used 60 units of slow-acting insulin each morning and evening and 5–8 units of fast-acting insulin at each meal.

Her blood tests showed that her long-term blood sugar was far too high, even though she produced plenty of insulin herself (high C-peptide) and used approximately 150 units of insulin each day. The high insulin level was the reason for her weight gain, because insulin is a potent fat-storage hormone which also hinders fat metabolism. I was therefore interested in Mari discontinuing the use of insulin in order to make her weight loss easier. Her liver test for ALAT was too high, she was producing antibodies against her thyroid gland (anti-TPO antibodies) and had a low level of vitamin D (see pages 285, 287 and 289). At that time, her weight was 117.4 kilograms (18 stone 7) and her BMI 37.9. Despite four medications for high blood pressure, it was far too high, 180/95 mm Hg.

I asked Mari to gradually eat fewer carbohydrates in parallel with keeping a diary of her food consumption, blood sugar values and insulin doses. I explained carefully that she had to gradually reduce the insulin doses as she gradually reduced the carbohydrates. I recommended she take vitamin and mineral supplements. After four weeks, beaming with joy, she reported that she had managed to do without fast-acting insulin, and in addition she had reduced her use of long-acting insulin by five units in the morning and five units in the evening. Her blood sugar had been stable at 7–8 mmol/L. Her weight had been reduced by three kilograms (6.6 pounds) without even having to try. For further weight reduction, I recommended that Mari start with a low carb VLCD (see page 232), as it would then be easier for me to help her with the gradual reduction of insulin.

We exchanged many text messages while she was on the VLCD, because I wanted to assure myself that her blood sugar was under control and that she was gradually reducing her insulin doses. After four weeks on this diet, she reported that her blood sugar had stabilised between 6 and 7 mmol/L. Her weight had been reduced by another 5 kilograms (11 pounds), a total of 8 kilograms (1 stone 4) in two months. Her blood pressure had fallen to 140/80 mm Hg, and her muscle and joint pain had been reduced significantly. Mari had also become slimmer in her legs and had less fluid in her fingers. Her stomach was functioning as it should, and her energy had begun to come back. She had a desire to eat more regular food instead of the VLCD products, and I explained to her carefully that she had to limit her carbohydrate consumption to 20–30 grams per day and eat mostly meat, poultry, fish, shellfish, eggs, dairy products without added sugar, avocado, nuts and vegetables. After another five weeks, she had quit using insulin. Her weight had been reduced by another 7 kilograms (1 stone 1), and she was extremely pleased.

After three months, Mari's long-term blood sugar had been reduced from 11.2 to 7.2 percent, at the same time as she had quit using insulin. Her own insulin production increased significantly when she quit using insulin injections; meaning that she had been very insulin resistant and needed a lot of insulin to keep her blood sugar under control. The values for ALAT and vitamin D had been normalised, and the anti-TPO value had been halved.

Weight loss went a little slower after a while, but even so Mari reduced her weight by 20 kilograms (3 stone 2) in five months. She continued the follow-up with her GP, who had been informed during the process about the treatment I was providing. The regular doctor gradually reduced her hypothyroid and blood pressure medications and had her in for check-ups regularly. Mari has understood that she must live on a low carb diet for the rest of her life but doesn't think it is any big sacrifice, seen in relation to all the positive effects of her new regime.

Blood test results before and after diet change.

Blood test	Before – with insulin	After 3 months – without insulin	Reference range
Long-term blood sugar (%)	11.2	7.2	< 6.1
C-peptide (pmol/L)	827	1600	< 700
Insulin (pmol/L)	547	-	18–173
ALAT (U/L)	72	38	< 45
Anti-TPO (kU/L)	164	79	< 35
Vitamin D_3 (nmol/L)	33	115	50–150

Gestational diabetes

Several studies have shown that women who have had gestational diabetes have a higher incidence of high blood pressure, diabetes and cardiovascular disease later in life than women who were healthy during their pregnancies.

Gall stones

During the last few decades, fat has been blamed for the formation of gall stones. This is not logical, as a lot of fat increases the excretion of bile and bile salts. More recent studies confirm, not surprisingly, that the greater the consumption of carbohydrates, the higher the risk is for the formation of gall stones.

Cardiovascular disease

Diabetics have a significantly increased risk of cardiovascular disease. This also applies to people with low sugar tolerance as established by a glucose tolerance test. Studies have shown that the lower the blood sugar is, the lower the risk of cardiovascular disease. This also applies within the normal range for fasting blood sugar and long-term blood sugar (HbA_{1c}).

Hypothyroidism (low metabolism)

Studies show that insulin resistance and metabolic syndrome (see pages 291 and 293) can be connected to disorders in the thyroid gland and hypothyroidism (see page 141). The most common cause for hypothyroidism is a chronic inflammation in the thyroid gland in which anti-TPO is shown in 80–90 percent of the cases. Anti-TPO are antibodies which attack and can damage the thyroid gland. In medical books, it is stated that anti-TPO is not affected by treatment with thyroxine, and that it is therefore not necessary to check this blood test. As you see in the table on the previous page, the value for anti-TPO was greatly reduced after Mari had eaten low carb food for three months.

Gunnar used insulin, gained weight and had neuralgia in his legs

Gunnar was 67 years old when he was referred to me from another doctor because he wanted to get better control over his diabetes. Gunnar's parents were healthy and lived to be very old, and he has two brothers who do not have diabetes. Gunnar had a sedentary occupation as a taxi driver and for a time ate a lot of fast food from petrol stations and kiosks. This food was rich in both carbohydrates and unnatural fats. Gunnar developed type 2 diabetes when he was 58 years old, and then he quit smoking for good. The same year, he developed a chronic colon inflammation. For the diabetes, he was first treated with metformin, but he had to quit using the medicine because of stomach pains and diarrhoea. The past four years, he had been forced to use insulin injections. He used both fast-acting and slow-acting insulin – in all, 270 units each day. He was often plagued with low blood sugar and ate high carbohydrate food in order to get it up again. At those times he had a tendency to eat too much, so that his blood sugar rapidly became too high. In addition to insulin, he was using nine other medications for high blood pressure, high cholesterol and chronic intestinal inflammation. Gunnar was often dizzy and always felt tired and weak, but his biggest problem was severe pain in his feet due to neuropathy. Neuropathy is a form of nerve damage which is common with diabetes and is due to excessive blood sugar over a long period. He slept poorly because of this pain and often took pain tablets without them helping much. He had to get up and urinate three times every night. In addition, his sexual potency was completely gone – a common complication with diabetes due to a low testosterone level and damage to the blood vessels

113

and/or the nerves. After he got diabetes, he ate a typical modern diet, including plenty of bread and potatoes, but very rarely any sweets. Gunnar wasn't able to exercise very much because of the pain in his feet.

His weight was 124 kilograms (19 stone 7) and his BMI 38. His blood pressure was 160/80 mm Hg, despite the fact that he was using three different blood pressure medications. Gunnar had a lot of fat around his stomach and excessive blood sugar, even though he used insulin. He was producing plenty of insulin (C-peptide) himself, but it worked very poorly because of the insulin resistance. His testosterone level was extremely low, and his levels of triglycerides, homocysteine and creatinine were too high (see pages 287, 281, 283 and 285).

Gunnar was willing to start a low carb VLCD (see page 232) in order to achieve rapid weight loss and to get good control of his carbohydrate consumption while he gradually reduced the insulin. We postponed the diet for three weeks because Christmas was close at hand. He reduced his weight by 1.8 kilograms (4 pounds) at Christmas just by being a little more careful with his consumption of carbohydrates. He came for a consultation after Christmas, and I told him how he should prepare the VLCD meals. I explained carefully how to reduce his insulin doses gradually as his blood sugar levels got lower. When he came for a check-up after three weeks, he reported that he had noticed, after just a few days, that he had less pain in his feet, but he still had diminished feeling in them. He had gradually reduced his insulin doses. He was 7.4 kilograms (1 stone 2) lighter and had only been using 30 units of insulin in the evening. He had become more energetic, his dizziness had disappeared, he slept better and felt very good. His blood sugar had been between 7 and

9 mmol/L, which was still a little too high but acceptable in a transitional phase. His blood pressure had fallen to 140/80 mm Hg. I encouraged him to go on walks and to start some careful strength training at home. Exercising with weights is very effective for keeping blood sugar down, because the muscles take up and break down sugar both during the heavy work and for a long time after training has stopped. We agreed that Gunnar should replace one powder meal with meat or fish and vegetables and not to take insulin if his blood sugar was below 9 mmol/L.

After another four weeks, he came for a check-up and proudly reported that he had walked 30 minutes every day and, in addition, had begun to lift weights with some old dumbbells he had at home. He had used only 90 units of fast-acting insulin in the course of these four weeks. His weight had gone down another 4.1 kilograms (9 pounds), and he wished to continue having four powder meals and a low carb dinner for another month.

At the next check-up, he said that he needed the pills for acid reflux less frequently. His feet had improved each day, and his bowels also functioned much better than before. His weight had gone down by another 4.5 kilograms (10 pounds) for a total weight loss of 16.8 kilograms (2 stone 9). I advised Gunnar to introduce yet another meal with low carb foods, since he had quit using insulin and had control of his blood sugar.

After three months, the pains in his legs was completely gone, but he still had some reduced sensitivity in his feet. His blood pressure had fallen to 130/70 mm Hg, and his weight had gone down another 3.3 kilograms (7 pounds). His blood tests had become considerably better, even though they still weren't entirely optimal.

Gunnar gradually replaced the powder meals with low carb foods and more fat, and the weight loss continued. In the course of five months, he reduced his weight by 26 kilograms (4 stone 1). His long-term blood sugar, as measured by his GP, was 6 percent after six months, which is considered normal. In his application to renew his driving licence, he wrote that he no longer used insulin. The county medical officer figured this could not be true, and I had to write a physician's declaration to confirm that Gunnar's blood sugar values were fine without using insulin and that he was also rid of the neuropathy.

Blood test results before and after diet change.

Blood test	Before – with insulin	After 3 months – without insulin	Reference range
Long-term blood sugar (%)	7.6	7.3 (6.0 after 5 months)	< 6.1
C-peptide (pmol/L)	2640	1107	< 700
Insulin (pmol/L)	260	131	18–173
Homocysteine (µmol/L)	21.9	16.9	5–17
Triglycerides (mmol/L)	2.04	1.40	< 1.7
Testosterone (nmol/L)	5	7	8–35
Creatinine (µmol/L)	106	91	60–105

Creatinine

Creatinine is a measurement of kidney function, and elevated values mean reduced kidney function, which is common among patients with advanced diabetes.

Testosterone

Most people with type 2 diabetes are overweight and produce a lot of insulin. Many inject insulin below the skin as well. Insulin stimulates enzymes which transform testosterone to oestrogens in men. This means, among other things, that the testosterone level sinks. A low testosterone level results in more feminine features such as increased breast tissue and lowered sexual desire. Viagra and similar tablets do not, unfortunately, increase testosterone levels, but can get the blood vessels in the penis to expand, increasing the possibility of having sexual intercourse. Losing weight and reducing insulin production (by eating fewer carbohydrates) do, however, result in higher testosterone levels. It can, therefore, be a good idea to measure his testosterone level when a man is overweight and wants to lose weight. This can be the motivation he needs, because most men want a high testosterone level.

How to reduce the risk of getting type 2 diabetes

The most important thing you can do is to reduce your consumption of carbohydrates. This applies particularly to sugary foods like chocolate, buns, cakes and soda, but also starchy foods like bread, rice, pasta and potatoes, and fruits with high sugar content like grapes, bananas, figs and dried fruit. If you eat high carb grain foods, you ought to choose those that cause the lowest possible blood sugar increase. Examples of these are whole grain bread, wholemeal pasta and brown rice. Limit your fruit consumption to one piece of fruit per day and eat more berries and vegetables instead. Reduce your consumption of potatoes and other root vegetables and eat more natural fat and proteins.

Saturated fat is not dangerous if you eat few carbohydrates. You use it as fuel, and it does not effect the insulin secretion from the pancreas. Animal fats rarely contain more than 50 percent saturated fatty acids and do not constitute any real danger, although one study has shown that a unilateral replacement of unsaturated fatty acids with saturated fatty acids resulted in increased insulin resistance. The reason for this is not necessarily the fat itself; it may also be due to fat-soluble toxins that can affect insulin sensitivity. Fat from dairy products (which contain about two-thirds saturated fatty acids) has been shown in several studies to *reduce* the risk of heart attack, despite that fact that it can increase the cholesterol in the blood. Even though natural coconut fat consists almost entirely of saturated fatty acids, several thousand years' use in Polynesia and other Southern Hemisphere countries has shown that it does not contribute to heart disease, obesity or diabetes when it is included in a diet that gives only small fluctuations in blood sugar. Coconut fat contains a large proportion of medium-length, saturated fatty acids that have beneficial health effects.

Because it is so important to avoid obesity, you should think about getting help to lose your excess weight. Obesity is caused, first and foremost, by a diet that contains a large proportion of high carb foods combined with fat. Regular exercise is important, particularly if you eat wrongly, because it will increase your tolerance of high carb foods. Chronic stress increases the secretion of cortisol from the adrenal glands, which contributes to increasing blood sugar and breaks down muscle mass. This, in turn, leads to a decrease in the body's ability to burn carbohydrates. Fluctuating blood sugar levels from eating a lot of high carb foods increases the body's production of stress hormones. In this way, eating the wrong food can also increase stress on the body.

Fluctuating blood sugar

Diffuse symptoms and low blood sugar

The symptoms that a great many patients present to their doctors and other therapists are diffuse. They are examined with advanced techniques, and in many cases nothing wrong is discovered. They are often adviced to work less, take sleeping pills or "happy pills", to exercise and drink plenty of water, whereas some go on indefinite sick leave. The patients try to follow this advice, but for many there is no effect. Often, the explanation can be something so simple as low or rapidly falling blood sugar after meals or snacks.

For those who do not use diabetes medication, the major cause of low blood sugar is too many carbohydrates in the diet. When the condition is recurring, their quality of life is significantly reduced. It may sound strange that eating lots of carbohydrates can result in low blood sugar, but here's the explanation:

High consumption of carbohydrates leads to rising blood sugar, which leads to a lot of insulin being released into the blood. The insulin signals for the sugar to be transported into the cells. Some people produce too much (or are particularly sensitive to) insulin, so that more sugar than necessary enters the cells. The result becomes rapidly falling or low blood sugar. If foods containing sugar or starch are consumed to help the situation, even more insulin is produced.

The episodes with low blood sugar continue, and the condition often worsens over time. Eating more carbohydrates when you have problems with low blood sugar can be compared to substance abusers who continue to take the substance every time they experience abstinence, in order to make themselves feel better. In the long run, substance abusers should gradually reduce the amount they take; then their withdrawal symptoms would disappear. The same principle applies to people who suffer from low blood sugar.

Common symptoms of rapidly falling or low blood sugar

1. Dizziness
2. Fainting
3. Spasm
4. Headache/migraine
5. Unclear vision
6. Concentration difficulties
7. Impaired memory
8. Woolly-headed feeling
9. Cold hands and feet
10. Numbness
11. Excessive sweating
12. Sleep disturbances
13. Heart palpitations
14. Uneasiness
15. Anxiety
16. Stomach cramps
17. Obesity

When blood sugar falls rapidly, the brain functions poorly, resulting in the symptoms listed in points 1–8. The body tries to get the blood sugar up again by producing several hormones such as growth hormone, glucagon, cortisol, noradrenaline and adrenaline. The effects of adrenaline are felt particularly strongly. See symptoms 9–16. Low blood sugar triggers a feeling of hunger and particulary a need for something sweet. This often results in frequent consumption of sweets and thereby weight gain.

Traditional medical treatment
of low blood sugar (reactive hypoglycaemia)

For those diagnosed, an ordinary high carb diet is recommended with frequent, small, and high fibre meals.

Kristine didn't feel well

Kristine was 40 years old when she came to me. She was plagued by long-lasting chills, dry skin, headaches, dizziness, insomnia, inner anxiety, mood swings, a bloated stomach, constipation, a craving for sweets and a total lack of energy. All these health problems diminished her quality of life considerably. She didn't understand what was wrong, as she was in fact eating healthy food and exercising regularly.

She had been to her GP with these problems. She was prescribed sleeping pills and told to exercise. Kristine took the pills and exercised more without getting any better.

When we first met, she told me that she had had border-line high blood sugar during her last pregnancy, and that she had put on 6 kilograms (13 pounds) in the last few years. She had two children in primary school and a part-time job. Kristine didn't think she had a lot of work pressure but, nonetheless, always felt worn out and stressed. Her breakfast consisted of caffè latte with extra-low fat milk, fruit yogurt, and two cups of fresh-pressed juice that she made herself. For lunch, she ate two slices of bread with meat, fish or cheese, and for dinner, meat, fish or chicken with potatoes, rice or pasta and plenty of vegetables. In the evening she had a strong craving for sweets, which she satisfied by eating a little dark chocolate or ice cream. She allowed herself this because she had never had weight problems. In addition, she drank a little tea with honey.

Based on her case history and diet, the diagnosis was simple to make. She was suffering from reactive hypoglycaemia, also called low blood sugar. All her blood tests were normal, and she had a BMI of 24. In other words, she was of normal weight. I explained carefully to her the relationship between her diet and the reactions she was having and advised her to eat three main meals and two small meals in-between. For breakfast, I suggested that she exchange fruit juice and yogurt with a slice of dark rye bread with butter and plenty of meat or fish, or a low carb muesli – in other words, few grains and sweet fruit but lots of nuts and seeds. For lunch, I recommended an omelette with vegetables as a side dish, and for dinner I would prefer that she eat far less rice, potatoes and pasta and instead increase the amount of vegetables. For "in-between" meals, I suggested nuts, or nuts plus a piece of fruit; alternatively cottage cheese with a few berries, half an avocado, some bits of cheese or crisp bread with something high in protein or fat on it.

Kristine returned after four weeks and reported that she had felt better after just a few days on the new diet. She fell asleep easily and slept the whole night. The uneasiness and stress in her body had disappeared, and her stomach and bowels functioned normally and she was no longer bloated.

In addition, her headaches and dizziness had gone away, and her energy and good humour had returned. The craving for sweets in the evening disappeared, and as a bonus she quickly lost the 6 kilograms (13 pounds) that had sneaked up on her in the last few years.

Treatment of low blood sugar

- Gradually reduce your consumption of carbohydrates to 50–70 grams per day.
- When you eat fewer carbohydrates, you have to eat more fat and possibly a little more protein.
- Increase your consumption of fat from oily fish (salmon, trout, mackerel, sardines and herring).
- Consume greater amounts of nuts, seeds, cold-pressed oils, avocados, cheese, butter, cream, sour cream and crème fraîche.
- Vary your protein sources with different types of meat and fish, eggs, cottage cheese and other cheeses.
- If you don't like to eat large portions or a lot of fat, I recommend three main meals and two "in-between" meals. Three meals are enough if you eat larger portions or plenty of fat. The more carbohydrates you eat, the greater the need will be for "in-between" meals because of the blood sugar fluctuation.
- The carbohydrates you eat should mainly be of a type that gives the least possible blood sugar increase. Examples are whole grain bread, low carb bread, wholewheat pasta and brown rice.
- Carbohydrates should be eaten together with protein and/or fat. This reduces the blood sugar increase and, subsequently the secretion of insulin from your pancreas.

- Eat for example fruit together with nuts or cottage cheese, natural yogurt or cream.

Magne was on sick leave because of dizziness

Magne was 60 years old when his GP referred him to me because of dizziness. The GP wondered if this had something to do with his blood sugar, since his long-term blood sugar was too high. He had also referred him for various brain tests at the hospital.

Magne was so dizzy that he couldn't manage to work and had been on sick leave for a long time. He also told me that it felt as though he had "fog" in his head. He ate regular food that included grain products, fish, meat, eggs, and a lot of fruit and vegetables. He cared little about sweets and potato crisps. He used medication for high blood pressure and high cholesterol, in addition to blood-thinning medications. Magne had repeatedly been shown to have too much ferritin in his blood, but there was no-one in the family with haemochromatosis (a genetically-predisposed disease caused by elevated iron absorption. Based on Magne's symptoms and his slightly elevated long-term blood sugar, I figured that fluctuating blood sugar was the problem. I therefore advised him to eat much fewer carbohydrates and more fat and protein.

When he returned after four weeks, he said that he was eating considerably less bread, potatoes, rice, pasta and fruit. He felt much better already after the first day on the new diet, and he was soon back his good old self again. His dizziness and the "fog" in his head had disappeared within a couple of days. The blood tests taken before the dietary changes showed that the values for C-peptide (955 pmol/L), long-term blood sugar (6.1 percent), ferritin (445 µg/L) and ALAT (80 U/L) were too high. Fasting blood sugar was in the boundary range (5.9 mmol/ L). In Norway, the experts have defined a fasting blood sugar between 4 and 6 mmol/L as normal, while everything over 6 mmol/L is called a high fasting blood sugar. The American Diabetes Association operates with a lower boundary, and it has defined a fasting blood sugar over 5.6 mmol/L as high.

Using a particular calculation, I could tell Magne that his high ferritin level was not due to the hereditary condition haemochromatosis. Actually, high ferritin levels are very common in people with insulin resistance and diabetes, without there being excessive iron in the blood. The cause of this is probably an inflammation in the body. Magne's high insulin level a good enough explanation, because too much insulin promotes inflammation.

Magne felt that all his physical problems were solved, and cancelled the tests he had been scheduled for at the hospital. He wanted, quite simply, to continue with the low carb diet. I recommended some literature and follow-up visits with the GP to check on the discrepant blood test results.

Sugar dependency

What is sugar dependency?

Dependency is a pathological relationship with a mood-altering substance or activity with an expectation of a positive reward. Some of these substance are sugar, alcohol, nicotine and narcotics. People who easily become dependent often use substances which affect the brain, such as, alcohol and nicotine. Furthermore, it has been observed that alcoholics who stop drinking often start to use sugar as a mood-altering substance instead. No-one is born with sugar dependency, but American researchers believe that as many as 75 % are born with a hypersensitivity to sugar, and that 25 % of these are extremely sensitive.

In the Stone Age, there was a reason for being drawn to sugar, of which there was not much in nature. Because we lived as hunters and gatherers, it was important to eat sugar so that we could store energy for winter use, in the same way as the grizzly bear stores energy by eating sweet berries. The problem today is that we have far too much access to carbohydrates, which leads to the most sugar-sensitive among us having problems with limiting themselves. Not all people who are hypersensitive develop dependency; psychology and environmental factors are also an important part of the picture. The reason that some become dependent on some substances and others do not, has not been explained entirely. Some researchers claim that dependent individuals have too little of some signal substances in the brain.

Most people know that food containing sugar can provide quick energy. But this doesn't apply only to typical sweets like soda, fruit drinks, chocolate and cakes. It also applies to foods high in starch like bread, potatoes, rice and pasta. In addition, fat is often substituted with starch and sugar in low fat products. So if they contain less fat, they often contain more carbohydrates. It's claimed that sugar can be just as addictive as narcotics. If you're genetically pre-disposed to sugar addiction, the "high" effect from sugar is extra strong, but the effect soon passes. When the effect slows, you need more – and if you don't get it, you experience withdrawal symptoms in the form of mood swings, headaches and rest-lessness.

Being sugar-dependent means having a strong craving for high carb foods. The sugar provides a good feeling in the brain, but it also leads to large fluctuations in blood sugar. This results in symptoms that make it necessary to continue eating more carbohydrates. The sugar lays "tracks" in the brain that are difficult to get rid of. When experiencing falling blood sugar caused from a large secretion of insulin, many people have symptoms such as uneasiness, anxiety, perspiration and heart palpitations. Eating foods that con-tain sugar and starch reduces the symptoms, but the whole process will only repeat itself. In many cases, the depend-ency leads to sequelae – or secondary ailments – such as overweight, insulin resistance and type 2 diabetes.

As with all dependency, the only solution is to quit using the addictive substance. My experience is that many sugar-dependent people manage to do so when they get help in making dietary changes and stabilising their blood sugar.

Those who have the greatest problems also need psychological help.

Traditional medical treatment of sugar dependency

Dependency on sugar does not exist as a medical diagnosis. Nor do guidelines exist for doctors as regards treatment of this condition.

Irene was addicted to sugar and thought she had a heart disease

Irene was 44 years old when a friend recommended she come to me because she had put on 20 kilograms (3 stone 2) in a relatively short time. She had tried innumerable diets but had discovered that nothing worked. Her weight stayed the same regardless of what she tried, and she was plagued by an enormous feeling of hunger. She ate a lot of bread in order to feel full, but she became hungry again shortly afterwards. She was out of condition; she felt drained of energy; her body was heavy and she had water retention in her hands and feet. Irene struggled hard when dieting but gave up quickly because she felt worn out and weak. Her willpower was at rock bottom, and she felt that she was no longer herself. She felt old and worn out, and became stressed and out of breath from the smallest exertions.

Irene was often plagued by heart palpitations and cold sweats, which scared her to death because she thought there was something seriously wrong with her heart. She was examined by a heart specialist, who found nothing wrong on the stationary bicycle test, ultrasound examination nor the heart rhythm monitor lasting several days. Irene's mood fluctuated greatly, she was seen as crabby and negative, she felt irritated and constantly got into arguments with family and colleagues. She often used food for comfort, and would always feel better after eating food that was high in carbohydrates, but she quickly became listless again. This resulted in her constantly putting something in her mouth without her being hungry. For breakfast she ate spelt bread and drank caffeine-free coffee on recommendation from the heart specialist. For snacks she often ate sweets because she "just had to." For lunch she also ate spelt bread or rice and beans. On the way home from her job, she often ate a chocolate bar or two because she hungered for sugar. For dinner there were various dishes with rice, beans or pulses and meat. Irene rarely ate fish. In the evening, she had an intense hunger for sweets and ate whatever chocolate, biscuits and the like she came across. If she didn't have sweets in the house, she ate slices of bread and fruit. She often woke during the night and couldn't get to sleep again before she had eaten bread, fruit or other high carb food.

I advised her to cut out all sweets and then to reduce her consumption of both bread and fruit. When she came for a check-up after four weeks, she said that she hadn't followed my advice entirely but had felt better the days she had been "smart". At times she ate a lot of chocolate. I explained to her yet again the connection between what she ate and her symptoms and said that she was a "chocoholic", with which she agreed. She was willing to try again, even though she felt that this was really difficult. We went through the blood tests, which showed that she had an excessive level of C-peptide and an insufficient level of vitamin D. It was in the middle of winter, so I recommended a vitamin D supplement in tablet form. The fact that she had insulin resistance was a strong motivator for making a better attempt over the next few weeks, since both her mother and aunt had diabetes.

After another four weeks, she reported proudly that she hadn't touched chocolate. Actually, she had cut out nearly all carbohydrates apart from vegetables and nuts. She had experienced withdrawal symptoms the first few days in the form of headaches and uneasiness, but fortunately it abated. She felt good, and her energy had returned. At the next check-up, Irene said that she had gotten heart palpitations one day after she had eaten some fruit. I told her that she was very sensitive to sugar and that she must always eat fruit together with a little fat in order to avoid these symptoms. Blood tests taken after six months showed a great improvement, and as a bonus she had reduced her weight by 12 kilograms (1 stone 13) without having felt that she was on a diet.

Blood test results before and after diet change.

Blood test	Before	After 6 months	Reference range
C-peptide (pmol/L)	964	758	< 700
Vitamin D_3 (nmol/L)	18	93	50–100

Individual carbohydrate tolerance in sugar-sensitive people

I see many patients who have gained weight because of sugar dependency. They come to me because they want to lose weight and learn to eat properly. Many of these patients get rid of their problems, to their great surprise, when they get their blood sugar stabilised by eating low-carb food. If they try to eat sweets again, they quickly notice that the craving for sweets and the need to cheat returns. Many understand that it's easier to avoid such temptations. Most can satisfy themselves with 70 % chocolate, but a few have a need for more sweet foods. How many grams of carbohydrates can be tolerated before the craving for sweets appears is individual. One must try out different foods in order to discover one's own limits.

Eating disorders

What are eating disorders?

The best-known eating disorders are anorexia, bulimia and overeating. A person has an eating disorder when the thoughts, feelings and behaviour of a person about food, body and weight, start to limit their self-realisation and impair their quality of life. These disorders can develop differently for different people. Some almost stop eating, hide food away and think they look very good, even though others tell them that they do not look healthy. Some alternate between not eating and then eating a lot. Some plan large intakes of food with subsequent vomiting or use of powerful laxatives.

Eating disorders are classified as psychological disorders in official diagnosis systems, because it's thought that a person with eating disorders also has difficulties in relation to his or her own thoughts and feelings. But of course, one can ask – which came first, the chicken or the egg? People who overeat and vomit have difficulties in any event with their own thoughts and feelings. They feel that they don't have control over themselves, their self-esteem is nil, they're ashamed and often have a guilty conscience. The question is why they have such big problems with food. My experience is that many of these patients can become healthy when they eat low carb food and have stable blood sugar. This also applies to sugar-dependent people, as demonstrated by Irene's history.

Traditional medical treatment of eating disorders

The cornerstones of treatment are empathy, motivation, guidance and monitoring. The goal is behavioural change.

Elisabet suffered from eating disorders for many years

Elisabet was 40 years old when she consulted me because she was struggling with her weight. She thrived best weighing 65 kilograms (10 stone 3), but her weight had gradually gone up to 80 kilograms (12 stone 8). Already from the time she was 14 years old, she had suffered from an eating disorder that resulted in her overeating and throwing up. The overeating involved unhealthy foods such as ice cream, chocolate and potato crisps. This usually occurred in the evening, and those closest to her didn't know that she was throwing up. At other times, she ate almost nothing. Elisabet alternated between bulimia and anorexia, which is quite common among those who have eating disorders. After dietary instruction from a nutritionist, she had managed better for a while, but now her eating was out of control again. Because she had good self-insight, she had tried treatment with a psychologist and a psychiatrist, without much success. An attempt with the pharmaceutical Reductil, which can reduce the interest in food, had no effect either.

I advised her to try a ketogenic diet with a consumption of 30–40 grams of carbohydrates per day – not primarily to lose weight, but because this could reduce her craving for sweets and other treats. She went along with this, and after two weeks she came for a check-up. She reported that she had been weak the first week, but then she started to feel very good, got more energy, and the craving for sweets disappeared entirely. To her great delight, she had also reduced her weight by 2.6 kilograms (5.7 pounds) in the course of these two weeks. The scale I use showed that 2.1 kilograms (4.6 pounds) of this was fat while 0.5 kilogram (1 pound) was water. Her blood tests were normal.

Elisabet started to go on long walks and felt very good. After another four weeks, she had lost another 1.2 kilograms (2.6 pounds) – a total of 3.8 kilograms (8.4 pounds) in six weeks. This is very good for a woman who, at the outset, had a BMI of 28. The most important thing for Elisabet, however, was that she felt completely cured of her eating disorder so long as she followed her new diet. She looked at me with big eyes and asked whether she could eat this way her whole life. I answered yes, of course, and added that she could increase her carbohydrate consumption to about 50 grams per day. I made it clear that it was good for her to eat a varied diet that included fish, shellfish, poultry, meat, eggs, unsweetened dairy products, cold-pressed oils, vegetables, berries, nuts, seeds and a little fruit. When consuming fruit and berries, it's good to eat proteins and fat at the same time, in order to reduce the increase in blood sugar. I pointed out how important it is to eat balanced meals that contain both protein, fat and a few carbohydrates.

Elisabet eventually lost som of her appetite and was given recipes and tips for preparing food. She introduced protein plates with added sweetener but quickly noticed that she got a sweet craving from them. I recommended a piece of fruit or nuts instead, and this satisfied her need.

Brita had an eating disorder and developed diabetes

Brita was 50 years old when she came to me because she wanted to lose weight. She felt that the task was impossible and that she needed help. When she was younger, she had suffered from a serious eating disorder in which she had alternated between anorexia and bulimia. She had been admitted to hospital for a period because her weight had been as low as 35 kilograms (5 stone 7). Her problem more recently had been a great craving for sweets, and she ate a lot of unhealthy food in order to meet this strong need. She often woke during the night and could put away large quantities of chocolate, biscuits and cakes before she finally fell asleep again. Her weight only increased, and none of her clothes fit her any longer. Everything had become an effort, she was always tired and she completely lacked energy. Brita went regularly to a doctor because she had high blood pressure and a high cholesterol level, for which she used medicines. There were many people in Brita's family who were seriously overweight, especially on her mother's side. They had slim legs but a lot of fat on the upper body. Her mother's mother and three of her aunts had type 2 diabetes, and two of them used insulin injections in order to control their blood sugar.

Brita weighed 118 kilograms (18 stone 8), had a BMI of 43. Her blood pressure was too high (150/85 mm Hg) despite use of two blood pressure medications. She received both verbal and written information about what she should eat in the time ahead. I advised her to cut out all the sweets first and then gradually reduce starchy foods such as bread, potatoes, rice and pasta.

Brita came for a check-up after four weeks. She had understood the message well and had cut out nearly all her carbohydrates, even though I had suggested a gradual reduction. I was impressed by her effort; Brita told me that she was a person who finished things she started. In addition, she had carefully considered everything I had explained to her and found it very logical and understandable. To her great delight, her craving for sweets had completely disappeared. She had been bothered by leg cramps, but otherwise the transition to the new diet had gone well, and she felt very good. She slept much better and was in better shape. Her weight was 8 kilograms (1 stone 4), and her blood pressure had normalised, that is to say 120/70 mm Hg. The blood tests that were taken before the dietary changes showed that she had excessive levels of C-peptide, sugar, uric acid, homocysteine, ALAT and creatinine and insufficient levels of SHBG and vitamin D. I recommended a vitamin D supplement in the form of tablets.

Brita became frightened when I told her that she had developed type 2 diabetes. She thought of her grandmother, who had been plagued by this disease. I told her that if she managed to continue with the new diet, her blood sugar would normalise, and as an extra bonus, she would lose more weight. The thought of her grandmother's suffering further motivated her to continue with this diet. She was willing to try everything to avoid diabetes. I advised her to continue with a ketogenic diet and supplements of vitamins, minerals and fatty acids. I explained to her that the leg cramps were due to a loss of salt and that it was important that she took the dietary supplements I recommended to her.

After eight weeks, Brita had reduced her weight by another 5 kilograms (11 pounds) and was very pleased. She said that in the last week she had felt foggy after breakfast and had experienced some flashes of light. I asked her what she had been eating for breakfast recently. Oatmeal cooked with water, she said. She had previously been eating omelettes, so I advised her to start again. I explained that the symptoms could be due to low or rapidly falling blood sugar. After having eaten carbohydrate-rich breakfast, her body produced a lot of insulin, with rapid decrease in blood sugar as a result. The leg cramps disappeared after she started with the dietary supplements.

After 12 weeks, her weight had gone down another 7 kilograms (1 stone 1), and her total weight loss was 20 kilograms (3 stone 2). The symptoms after breakfast had disappeared after she started eating omelettes. Her mood and breathing had become much better. She had felt a strong need to move about and now went on a two-hour walk every day. She felt that she had got her life back and became very happy when she saw how good her blood tests had become. Brita continued with the low carb diet and adjusted to it well. I advised her to double the vitamin D dosage, since the level in her blood was still too low.

After six months, Brita had reduced her weight by 35 kilograms (5 stone 7) and felt like a 30-year-old again. She gradually increased her carbohydrate consumption slightly, but she still lost another five kilograms (11 pounds) over a few months. When she reached 75 kilograms (11 stone 11) and had a BMI of 28, both she and I felt that the goal had been achieved. Her actual goal was 60 kilograms (9 stone 6), but we agreed that it wouldn't be particularly attractive after the great weight loss. Losing 35 kilograms (5 stone 7) leaves a lot of excess skin, and then there's no point in being as thin as a sylph. The most important goal for Brita was to continue with the low carb diet and maintain her weight.

Blood test results before and after diet change.

Blood test	Before	After 3 months	Reference range
Blood sugar (mmol/L)	7.4	5.7	4–6
C-peptide (pmol/L)	1349	971	< 700
SHBG (nmol/L)	15	27	23–100
Gamma GT (U/L)	139	88	11–77
Uric acid (µmol/L)	432	364	155–400
Creatinine (µmol/L)	97	89	50–90
Vitamin D_3 (nmol/L)	28	41	50–150
Homocysteine (µmol/L)	17.0	13.4	4.0–15.4

Comfort eating

Karin Sveen's expression "Food is thin comfort – that's why there has to be so much" is striking and important. Some of my patients have an eating disorder in the form of comfort eating, which is not necessarily a medical diagnosis. This applies very often to women (with whom I have the most experience) who commit themselves to many responsibilities and have little time for themselves. They have a job, responsibility for the house and children along with elderly parents, parents-in-law and perhaps a sick friend. Their time goes to commuting between home, nurseries, schools, the children's leisure activities, rest homes, nursing homes and hospitals where they help, pick up, clean, comfort and encourage. Some of these people snack the entire time between all the tasks, and even though they eat little each time, their consumption of food becomes large in the course of the day. The food is often eaten on the run wherever there is food available. For the most part it involves quick fixes such as bread, buns, cakes, chocolate, sausages and slices of pizza. Others eat mostly in the evening, when they finally get a few minutes for themselves and feel that they deserve a reward after the day's hard work. They give and give the entire day, but often get little support, thanks and encouragement in return. Therefore they comfort and relieve themselves with food, preferably something sweet and fatty that calms the brain for a brief while. They know that it isn't healthy, that they're putting on weight and they have a guilty conscience – but they aren't able to stop. These women are constantly on diets and know almost everything about food, dieting and calories. When they do get round to dieting they usually lose 10 kilograms (1 stone 8), but they can't maintain focus on food or themselves and quickly gain the weight all over again.

Is this you? If so, try to find room for yourself! Everyone needs time for themselves – for reflection, exercise, friends, cultural experiences and the like. Seek a few nice experiences every day – life will become easier to live, and you won't need to alleviate all problems with sweets, alcohol or other substances that affect the brain. Say no now and then; you don't always have to be the one who always says yes and takes responsibillity for most everything. This can be difficult, as you have a guilty conscience when you say no, and a guilty conscience often leads to eating too much or eating the wrong things. But as you know – practise makes perfect. Start by telling the people who know you best what your new regime entails. Tell them that now you want to prioritise your own health, and that you need a little extra time for this. If you gain understanding for your plan, that's wonderful.

Many people feel, however, that they get verbal support, while nothing happens at the practical level. In this case, you must carry out what you have set yourself to do, and the people you surround yourself with can think what they like! Make a list of the week's duties and eliminate everything that is not completely necessary. Then you'll see that there's a great deal that doesn't have to be done that week.

If you cannot change your self-image and your behaviour pattern, you should get a referral to a professional counsellor, preferably together with your nearest relative(s). Everyone needs to be seen, heard and have physical contact.

Hypothyroidism

What is hypothyroidism?

Hypothyroidism means a low function of the thyroid gland. The popular term for hypothyroidism is low metabolism, but metabolism encompasses all chemical processes that occur in the cells in the body and is not controlled only by the thyroid gland. Two to three percent of the population are thought to have hypothyroidism. The most common cause is an inflammation which makes the body produce antibodies against the thyroid gland. These antibodies can be shown in the blood and are called anti-TPO. The thyroid gland lies at the front of the throat, just below the larynx. It produces thyroxine (T4) and a little triiodothyronine (T3). It's the pituitary gland in the brain which determines how much T4 and T3 are to be produced. The pituitary gland stimulates the thyroid gland with the help of a thyroid gland-stimulating hormone (TSH), so that more T4 and T3 are produced. If the production of T4 and T3 ceases for any reason, or if the hormones are working poorly, the pituitary gland sends out more TSH into the blood stream.

Thyroxine travels with the blood to all the cells in the body. Here T4 is converted into T3, which is five to six times more potent than T4 – but both increase the tempo of a great many of the chemical processes in the body. The diagnosis of hypothyroidism is usually made when TSH is too high and T4 is too low (that is to say, that the values are outside defined boundaries), but according to the American physician and researcher Mark Starr, one can suffer from hypothyroidism even if these measurements are normal. With hypothyroidism, symptoms can manifest from most organ systems. These symptoms develop gradually as a rule, so that a long time can pass before the individual, or their surroundings, react to something being wrong.

People with hypothyroidism commonly experience dry skin, dry hair with split ends, hair loss, brittle and thin nails, swelling around the eyes, hoarseness, constipation, joint pain, heart problems, sluggish movements, fatigue, increased need for sleep, depression, problems with concentration and memory, menstrual disorders, reduced sex drive, infertility and a tendency to be cold. Hypothyroidism often occurs simultaneously with other conditions where one's own immune defences are over-activated, such as type 1 diabetes, arthritis, coeliac disease and pregnancy. Hypothyroidism is not uncommon among women two to six months after delivery. Several patient case histories in this book show that patients who have hypothyroidism often have several other inflammatory conditions simultaneously.

Traditional medical treatment of hypothyroidism

Hypothyroidism that is due to disease in the thyroid gland is treated with thyroxine. The dosage is increased gradually until TSH has become normal.

Subclinical hypothyroidism

The term subclinical hypothyroidism is used for a condition where the patient doesn't have obvious physical signs of hypothyroidism but an elevated level of TSH is shown, while the level of FT4 is normal. This is frequently the case. In a large scale investigation in Norway, this condition has been found among 3.6 % of men and 4.8 % of women in all age groups. The condition is far more common with increasing age. In the age group over 80 years, 11.3 % of men studied and 8.2 % of women studied had subclinical hypothyroidism. Patients who have been shown to have subclinical hypothyroidism should take regular blood tests in order to check whether the condition is developing into hypothyroidism.

Some patients get treatment with thyroxine even though they don't have hypothyroidism. There are often patients who have symptoms that resemble hypothyroidism. Several studies have shown that these patients experience no effects from taking thyroxine. The cause must therefore be something else, and thus we have to look a little closer at whether insulin can play a role.

Sugar, insulin and hypothyroidism

Many people who gain weight think there is something wrong with their metabolism, and thus they often think of the thyroid gland. The significance of hypothyroidism when it comes to weight gain is exaggerated, however. Metabolism is, moreover, far more than just the function of the thyroid gland. Metabolism includes many chemical reactions that occur in the cells and which are the basis for all life. Metabolism principally involves making use of nutrients – mostly carbohydrates, proteins and fats that are used for tissue formation and the production of energy – and removal of waste products. Metabolism is therefore divided into anabolism (building up) and catabolism (breaking down). Several hormones are important when it comes to metabolism, and as you have read earlier in the book, insulin plays a central role. Most overweight people have insulin resistance, which means that they convert carbohydrates to fat instead of using them for energy. Symptoms which are seen with hypothyroidism and subclinical hypothyroidism are also common with fluctuating blood sugar, insulin resistance and diabetes.

The effects of insulin on the thyroid gland's hormones have not been completely explained, but one theory is that insulin is necessary for the conversion of T4 to T3. If insulin doesn't work because of insulin resistance, TSH will increase because of too little active T3. A study has shown that 19.5 % of those who suffer from serious obesity, that is to say people who have a BMI > 40, also have TSH values that indicate hypothyroidism in varying degrees. It was also shown that TSH has a greater correlation with the degree of insulin resistance than with the degree of overweight. This means that high levels of insulin and insulin resistance are related more to hypothyroidism than the obesity itself.

My experience is that many patients with subclinical hypothyroidism and hypothyroidism also have insulin resistance, obesity and diabetes. Subclinical hypothyroidism with only elevated TSH is often normalised with the use of a low carb diet, so that blood sugar and insulin are normalised in parallel with weight loss. Often I must gradually reduce the medication dosage when patients with hypothyroidism lose weight eating low carb food. If you have symptoms which resemble those that have been indicated for hypothyroidism, I recommend that you also have the fasting C-peptide in your blood measured. A value over 700 pmol/L combined with abdominal obesity indicates insulin resistance and can be the explanation for all the symptoms you have. With insulin resistance, the muscle and liver cells receive less glucose because of the insulin resistance, at the same time as the body does poorly at burning fat, because insulin inhibits fat metabolism. Many people feel that there is something wrong with their metabolism, and in that case this is often the cause. In these cases, the cells are actually starving because they have access to too little glucose and, in addition, they burn too little fat. I suspect that this is one of the reasons for the low energy level many of my patients have. Their metabolism of fat starts up again if the body gets what it needs – more fat and fewer carbohydrates. Many people have been on diets their whole lives, which also does something to their metabolism. It shuts way down and the body uses less of the available energy uses than if sufficient food were available.

Anne had low metabolism and weight problems

Anne was 45 years old when she sought me out because she had gained weight in recent years and had problems with digestion and urination in addition to a low metabolism, for which she was being treated. She weighed five kilograms (11 pounds) when she was born, lost weight rapidly after birth and had been thin far into her school years. As a child, she was diagnosed with multiple allergies. In adulthood, her normal weight had been 50 kilograms (7 stone 12); she was 160 centimetres (5 feet 3 inches) tall. When she was 31 years old, she put on 10 kilograms (1 stone 8) in the course of a month without having changed her lifestyle. She managed to normalise her weight again in the course of nine months. Many in her family had type 2 diabetes, and all except Anne were very tall. In her first pregnancy, she put on 11 kilograms (1 stone 10) within the first three months, and at the end of the pregnancy she weighed 85 kilograms (13 stone 5). Three months after the delivery, she was diagnosed with hypothyroidism and was treated with thyroxine. One year after the delivery, she had reduced her weight to 58 kilograms (9 stone 2) by going for a walk every day and eating frequent and small meals. Even though she followed the dietary advice recommended by health officials, her weight increased gradually to 85 kilograms (13 stone 5), this time without being pregnant. She managed to reduce her weight by approximately 10 kilograms (1 stone 8) by eating smaller meals and being more active.

When Anne came to me, she ate as follows: for breakfast, rolled oats with low-fat milk or a slice of wholewheat bread with white cheese. For lunch, she ate one or two slices of wholewheat bread with cheese and vegetables. Dinner was meat or fish, with potatoes and vegetables. She seldom ate between meals and exercised regularly twice a week. Because of constant airway infections, depression and loss of energy, she had been on sick leave from her job for one year and was now in a rehabilitation programme. Anne regularly went to psychiatrists, used an antidepressant, always felt tired and had diffuse pains in her whole body.

Anne now weighed 76.4 kilograms (12 stone) and had a BMI of 29.8. The blood tests showed that she had an excessive C-peptide value and that the fats in her blood were very unfavourable. The metabolic tests were normal, however, because she took thyroxine tables daily.

Anne wished to try a low carb diet (VLCD), that she had read about. After seven weeks, she came for a check-up and was happy with the result. Her weight hade gone down 8.4 kilograms (1 stone 5), and she thought the diet was tasty and easy to follow. Anne gradually replaced the VLCD meals with regular low carbohydrate food, and after three months she had reduced her weight by 13 kilograms (2 stone 1). She had, however, developed a problem with her urination. Whenever she felt that she had to go to the toilet, she had to get there immediately. I advised her to gradually reduce the thyroxine, and thus the urinary problems disappeared. After six months, she quit using thyroxine entirely and felt very good.

Blood tests taken after 12 months showed a solid improvement. Her triglycerides, however, had not been reduced, so I asked Anne to have the test checked by her regular doctor. She was very pleased with the results and did well on a diet with more fat and fewer carbohydrates. The metabolic tests were completely normal without thyroxine after 18 months.

Blood test results before and after diet change.

Blood test	Before – with thyroxine	After 12 months – without thyroxine	Reference range
C-peptide (pmol/L)	1010	481	< 700
Total cholesterol (mmol/L)	8.3	5.8	3.3–6.9
HDL cholesterol (mmol/L)	1.3	1.5	1.0–2.7
LDL cholesterol (mmol/L)	6.0	3.5	1.4–4.7
Triglycerides (mmol/L	2.28	2.33	< 1.7
TSH (mU/L)	1.2	7.3 (2.7 after 18 months)	0.2–4.0
FT_4 (pmol/L)	13.2	10.8 (13 after 18 months)	9–22

Chronic inflammations

What is a chronic inflammation?

An inflammation is most often a reaction to cell damage and is one of the most common biological reactions in the body. The causes can be strong heat, irritating substances locally, injuries, infection with bacteria or viruses. To protect itself against these effects, the immune system uses various attack cells and antibodies. Common symptoms of inflammation are heat, pain, redness, swelling and reduced function. Inflammations can occur in all of the body's tissues and organs.

A chronic inflammation arises, for example, when the immune system attacks the body's own cells. This can lead to many serious diseases, including type 1 diabetes, arthritis, and skin and connective tissue disorders. A high consumption of carbohydrates, too many omega-6 fatty acids, low consumption of antioxidants, little physical activity and smoking increase the risk of chronic inflammation.

Sugar, insulin and chronic inflammation

A series of studies shows that inflammation is the underlying cause of an increasing number of diseases. As for example, cardiovascular disease, rheumatoid arthritis, osteoarthritis, fibromyalgia, dementia and Alzheimer's disease. High blood sugar results in increased inflammation in the body both directly and indirectly because it increases the levels of insulin. A contributory cause for inflammation can be getting too little magnesium. Studies have shown that over-weight people consume less magnesium and have a lower magnesium level in the blood than people with normal weight. Magnesium plays an important role for insulin's effect in the uptake of sugar in the cells. In addition, insulin stimulates the uptake of magnesium in insulin-sensitive cells. If the cells are insulin resistant, the cells take up less mag-nesium. For this reason, insulin-resistant people should take more than official recommended dosage of magnesium. Imbalance in the consumption of polyunsaturated fatty acids is also of great significance in these diseases developing. Obesity is itself a common cause of chronic inflammation. Among other things, an increased production of markers for inflammation (for example CRP) is found in the fatty tissues of overweight people. It has been shown that a low carbo-hydrate diet reduces the concentration of CRP much more than a diet consisting of more carbohydrates and less fat.

My experience concurs with this. I advise my patients to eat far fewer carbohydrates and to increase their consump-tion of natural animal and vegetable fats. I advise many of them to take a magnesium supplement as well. The positive effects of this are that, in addition to weight reduction, very many get rid of eczema, psoriasis, tenosynovitis, joint and muscle pains and other chronic inflammatory conditions.

The balance between omega-3 and omega-6 fatty acids

Omega-3 and omega-6 fatty acids are called essential fatty acids because they are required in several functions in the body necessary for life. Since we cannot make them our-selves, we are required to eat them. These essential fatty acids can be converted to eicosanoids, a group of hormone-like substances that affect most of the body's cells and functions and also control other hormones. Two main groups of eicosanoids are produced, and both have important functions in the body. Problems arise when there is an imbalance in the relationship between the two. In most Western countries, the consumption of omega-6 fatty acids is far too high. Many people will therefore experience too many of the effects that you will find in the right hand column in the following table, and too few of those which are on the left.

Effects of eicosanoids that are created from omega-3 and omega-6 fatty acids.

Sufficient omega-3 fatty acids	Excessive omega-6 fatty acids
Counteracts sticky blood	Leads to more sticky blood
Expands the blood vessels	Constricts blood vessels
Reduces inflammation	Promotes inflammation
Reduces pain	Increases pain
Stimulates immune response	Suppresses immune response
Stimulates brain function	Suppresses brain function

Fibromyalgia

Fibromyalgia is a relatively new diagnosis in medicine, and in traditional medical environments it's said that the cause is unknown. It's assumed that long-term mental and physical overtaxing are significant. The condition is characterised as a pain syndrome consisting of a collection of symptoms. It is distinguished by chronic muscle pains in several parts of the body and painful, pressure-sensitive tender points. Many patients have had health problems as early as in childhood, and the condition often becomes more prevalent with age. About 3 % of the population is affected, and about 90 % of those diagnosed are women. Many people with fibromyalgia become eligible for disability pensions. Typical symptoms are aching and burning pains in muscles and in the muscle attachments around joints. Common symptoms are sleep disorders, mood swings, chills, headaches, numbness, a bloated feeling, vision disorders, the feeling of having a lump in the throat, mental stress, fatigue, exhaustion, depression, memory loss, tinnitus, anxiety, concentration difficulties, dizziness, nausea, upset stomach and frequent urination.

If you look a little closer at these symptoms, you will notice that they recur in many of the patient case histories I have recounted in the book. The question thus becomes whether the cause is so unclear – or can a good deal of the problems be explained by fluctuating blood sugar and high insulin production?

Traditional medical treatment of fibromyalgia

It's claimed that there is no curative medical treatment for fibromyalgia, and ordinary pain relief medicines have little effect. Measures which can alleviate it are physical training, treatment with medications that are used for depression, good information, behavioural therapy or a combination of such measures.

Eva had fibromyalgia and type 2 diabetes

Eva was 66 years old when she came to me because she wanted to lose weight. But it wasn't just her weight that was her problem. For ten years she had been plagued with strong muscle and joint pains and had been diagnosed with fibromyalgia. This bothered her day and night to such a degree that she had to use many pain relief tablets. Her quality of life was considerably reduced because of this disorder. Eva had also developed type 2 diabetes, for which she used two different medications, in addition to two drugs for high blood pressure. She always felt bloated and distended in her stomach, was plagued with acid reflux and used tablets daily to control her heartburn.

Her weight was 87.8 kilograms (13 stone 12) and her BMI 35.2. The blood tests showed that she had excessive levels of C-peptide, sugar and Micro-CRP, an insufficient level of SHBG and an unfavourable profile of fats. Eva wished to start a diet such as a VLCD with a low carbohydrate content in order to get a quick and motivating weight reduction. I explained to her that she had to quit using her blood-sugar lowering medication when she started with a VLCD, or she could end up with too low blood sugar.

When Eva came for a check-up after four weeks, she had reduced her weight by 6.3 kilograms (1 stone). She said with great enthusiasm that the muscle pains had disappeared completely after just one week. She had quit using her blood-sugar medication, and her blood sugar had been at 6–9 mmol/L, which is acceptable in this phase. I advised her to replace the one powder meal with a low carb meal consisting of meat or fish and vegetables that grow above the ground. After another four weeks, she had reduced her weight by another 2.7 kilograms (6 pounds) and felt very good. She was also breathing better. She was a little disappointed over the weight loss this time but was pleased when I explained to her that she had reduced her fat mass by 4.7 kilograms (10 pounds) and, for some reason, had gained two kilograms (4 pounds) of water. Her blood sugar had decreased even more and was between 6 and 7 mmol/L. In the course of five months, she reduced her weight by 13.6 kilograms (2 stone 2), and her blood tests were much better than when she started. She was extremely satisfied with this result and looked forward to buying new clothes.

Then came Christmas, and Eva didn't manage to maintain the low carb diet. She cheated with cakes, desserts and potatoes. She became stiffer in her body, breathed more heavily, put on 3 kilograms (6.6 pounds) and her blood pressure rose. When the muscle pain returned, she again cut down on her carbohydrate consumption, and her muscle pains disappeared. She was amazed that diet could mean so much for her body.

Blood test results before and after diet change.

Blood test	Before	After 5 months	Reference range
Blood sugar (mmol/L)	9.3	6.9	4–6
Long-term blood sugar (%)	8.6	6.1	< 6.1
C-peptide (pmol/L)	915	742	< 700
SHBG (nmol/L)	15	23	23–100
Triglycerides (mmol/L)	4.5	1.4	< 1.7
Total cholesterol (mmol/L)	7.5	6.0	3.9–7.8
HDL cholesterol (mmol/L)	1.4	1.5	1.0–2.7
Total/HDL cholesterol	5.4	4.0	< 4.0
LDL cholesterol (mmol/L)	4.7	4.2	2.0–5.3
Micro-CRP (mg/L)	5	3.4	<5

High blood sugar and fibromyalgia

There is a clear correlation between blood sugar values and fibromyalgia. A study has shown that 17 % of all the patients in a group with diabetes and just 2 % of the people in the group without diabetes had fibromyalgia. The diabetes patients who had the most serious fibromyalgia also had the highest long-term blood sugar (HbA1c).

Åse had fibromyalgia and inflammation in one arm

Åse was 50 years old when she came to me after a recommendation from her general practioner. She had always struggled with being overweight and was a yo-yo dieter. She had been diagnosed with fibromyalgia several years previously. Åse had had migraines for 25 years, but only every other month. When she had an attack, she had to lie down in a cold, dark room and was lucky if she slept it off. When she managed to get to bed in time, she avoided throwing up.

The main problem now was inflammation in one of her arms. Åse had sought out all possible therapists and had incurred great expenses without anything having helped. She had even been on sick leave for six months because of her arm. Åse had a typical modern diet but admitted that she probably ate too much cake, ice cream and chocolate. With a weight of 140.2 kilograms (22 stone 1) and a BMI of 44, she was diagnosed as morbidly obese. We agreed that Åse would first quit eating sweets and then gradually reduce other high carb foods over the course of one to two weeks. Afterwards, she would eat a ketogenic diet with just 20 grams of carbohydrates per day.

When Åse came for a check-up, she said that she had gradually reduced down to a ketogenic diet and that it had not been a problem. She noticed quickly that she had more energy and was in a better mood than before. She had reduced her weight by 7 kilograms (1 stone 1) during the first four weeks. Her craving for sweets had completely disappeared – now she could watch others eating cake without it tempting her in the least. Best of all, her arm was completely fine, and she didn't feel the fibromyalgia any longer. The blood tests that were taken before she changed diet showed that she had excessive levels of C-peptide and uric acid, but otherwise the tests were normal.

Åse continued with the low carb food and increased her activity level by going on short walks, in addition to doing simple exercises at home. After two months she had reduced her weight by another six kilograms (13 pounds). She felt very good and started at a part-time job. After yet another month, she started in a full-time position again and felt that she had got her life back. A check of the blood test analyses showed them to be completely normal. She felt that she was eating wonderful food, and that it was fun finding new recipes with few carbohydrates.

I had an e-mail from Åse one year after her dietary change, in which she reported that her weight had been reduced by 22 kilograms (3 stone 7) during the last year. The most important thing for her, however, was all the positive changes the low carb diet had led to. In Åse's words:

- I am very grateful that a name has been put to a problem I have struggled with my whole life.
- My self-respect has increased enormously – now it is me who has control over my body and not the other way around.
- I sleep better at night.
- My vision is clearer, and my eyes look healthier in colour.
- My stomach functions as it should. It is no longer bloated and distended.
- I haven't had a migraine or other headache in the last year.

- My tartar is as good as gone – my dentist thought this was very interesting.
- I have less fluid in my body, and my ankles have become slimmer.
- My skin is cleaner and more attractive.
- My body is "quicker" and more mobile and seems more flexible and less inflamed.
- I have less pain with menstruation.
- The hot flashes associated with menopause have diminished.
- My taste experiences are much better.

Blood test results before and after diet change.

Blood test	Before	After 2 months	Reference range
C-peptide (pmol/L)	1092	532	< 700
Uric acid (μmol/L)	444	357	155–400

Osteoarthritis

Osteoarthritis, also called arthrosis, is the most common rheumatic disease. It affects the back, hips, knees and fingers. More and more people all over the world are getting osteoarthritis, and at least 10 % of the population between 25 and 75 years old is presumed to have symptoms of the disease. Osteoarthritis occurs most frequently after the age of 45–50 and is characterised as an epidemic both in Norway and in the European Union. With osteoarthritis, the joint cartilage is damaged, so that bone rubs against bone in the joint cavity and the joints become stiff and painful. There is often reduced mobility in the joints and, with finger arthrosis, knots can often be seen on the middle and outer joints.

Traditional treatment of osteoarthritis

Pain-relieving medications are the usual treatment for osteoarthritis, but they don't remove the cause. Glucosamine can have a positive effect on the joint cartilage if the usual pain-relieving medicines do not have effect. For people of a certain age with severe osteoarthritis, a joint prosthesis is an alternative. Exercise, physiotherapy, a healthy diet according to official recommendations and maintaining a good weight are also recommended in medical guidelines.

Gunn had reduced quality of life because of osteoarthritis in both knees

Gunn was 53 years old when she sought me out because she wanted to lose weight. She had put on a lot of fat during her pregnancies, and in the course of her last pregnancy her weight had increased by as much as 30 kilograms (4 stone 10). She was constantly dieting and she had tried most diets without success. Gunn was very fond of chocolate and had a serious craving for sweets. Her father had a heart attack at 50, but no-one in the family had diabetes.

Gunn had been plagued for many years with pain in both her knees, and the X-ray images showed pronounced osteo-arthritis. She had become dependent on pain-relieving tablets both day and night. She often woke at night because of pain and was very troubled at work as well, where she had to stand and walk a great deal. In addition, she had pain in her muscles and finger joints.

Her weight was now 100 kilograms (15 stone 11) and her BMI 37. The blood tests showed that she had high Micro-CRP, a finding that fit well with her having osteo-arthritis. Having a lot of fat tissue results in increased inflammation, and inflammations often result in generalised pain in muscles and joints. In addition, increased inflammation in the body is an indicator of increased risk for cardiovascular disease. The other blood tests were normal, and C-peptide was < 700 pmol/L. Even though her C-peptide was relatively low, it was the hormone insulin which had made Gunn overweight. If high carb foods are eaten often, the insulin level will be high throughout the entire day, but it can fall to a normal value in the morning. With a continued high carb diet, the fasting C-peptide value will increase for most people.

I told Gunn how all this was connected and advised her first to gradually reduce her carbohydrate consumption. When she returned after four weeks, her craving for sweets had disappeared, and she had not been bothered by hunger as she had often been before. She was eager to lose weight, and so we started with a low carb diet (VLCD). I also recommended some vitamins, minerals and omega-3 fatty acids.

During the first five weeks, Gunn reduced her weight by 10 kilograms (1 stone 8), of which 8 kilograms (1 stone 4) were pure fat and two kilograms (4.4 pounds) were water. After another six weeks, she had lost another 6.5 kilograms (1 stone) and had begun to gradually reduce her intake of pain-relieving medicines. In the course of four-and-a-half months, she had reduced her weight by 22 kilograms (3 stone 7), was pain-free in her knees and managed without pain-relieving tablets. The blood tests she took after five months showed that her Micro-CRP was considerably reduced after the weight loss. Her C-peptide level was also reduced, even though it hadn't been particularly high at the outset. A lower consumption of carbohydrates leads to a reduction of the insulin level, and with that reduced inflammation.

When Gunn weighed 76 kilograms (12 stone) and had a BMI of 28, I referred her to a plastic surgeon because of the large flap of skin on her stomach after her great weight loss. She had surgery and was extremely pleased with the result. In Norway, the government pays for such operations, because having so much excess skin is seen as a medical problem. There are resulting problems such as soreness, fungal growth and bad odour when the skin lies in large folds on the belly. Skin can also be removed on the upper arms and thighs, and with a large loss of fat in the breasts, mammoplasty can be done. For many people, such an operation can function as a motivation for weight reduction. Seen from a socio-economic perspective, this is a small cost compared to the costs connected with all the diseases obesity can lead to.

Blood test results before and after diet change.

Blood test	Before	After 2 months	Reference range
Micro-CRP (mg/L)	10	3.9	< 4
C-peptide (pmol/L)	614	432	< 700

Bechterew's disease (Ankylosing Spondylitis)

Bechterew's disease is a chronic rheumatic disease of the connective tissue which usually affects the back, pelvis and rib cage. Jaw joints, shoulders, hips and knees may also be attacked. Many people get inflammations in their tendons, and the most common problems are pain and stiffness. Back stiffness is experienced most commonly after one has been at rest, especially in the morning. Pain in the night can be alleviated by standing up and moving about. The disease strikes most frequently among men between the ages of 18–40. Bechterew's disease is an autoimmune disease, that is to say that the body's immune response attacks its own tissue. Little is known about the causes of Bechterew's disease. A range of other conditions often accompany the disease that are not directly related to the inflammatory condition in the joints.

Traditional medical treatment of Bechterew's disease

The objective with the treatment is to reduce pain and stiffness, prevent dislocations in the skeleton, suppress the disease's activity and improve the patient's general quality of life. Pain-suppressing medications are used, and recently new pharmaceuticals have arrived which work on the disease process itself. Exercise, a healthy diet according to official recommendations, physiotherapy and residing in warm locations are also recommended.

Kari had Bechterew's disease and weight problems

Kari was 48 years old when she sought me out because she wanted to lose weight. She had had Bechterew's disease since she was 30 years old, and she had gotten infections in her eyes several times – which is a common secondary ailment. She was always tired and slept poorly. Her metabolic tests had been low in the reference range, and she had therefore received treatment with thyroxine. However, she hadn't felt better or got more energy taking this medication. She had to use pain-relieving tablets every day.

Kari ate a regular European diet with a lot of starchy food, but relatively few sweets. She worked out regularly at a fitness studio and also went on nature walks. Her weight had crept up over many years to 92 kilograms (14 stone 7), and this heaviness had begun to be a problem for her. Many in her family were plagued with obesity.

Her blood tests showed that she had excess levels of Micro-CRP, uric acid and triglycerides, while her C-peptide was not particularly high. We don't actually know what is an optimal value for C-peptide. Even with a normal C-peptide, too much sugar and insulin in the blood in the daytime can result in various problems, including weight gain, inflammation and loss of energy.

I advised Kari to quit eating sweets entirely and gradually reduce her intake of high carb foods such as potatoes, bread, rice and pasta. After one or two weeks she should only be eating approximately 20 grams of carbohydrates per day. I motivated her to cease eating grain products, because they can greatly promote inflammation due to, among other things, their high content of omega-6 fatty acids. When the consumption of carbohydrates is reduced in a regular diet, the consumption of fat must be increased. I advised Kari to eat a lot of oily fish, so that she would get plenty of omega-3 fatty acids.

Kari returned after four weeks and had reduced her fat mass by 2.7 kilograms (6 pounds). She had cheated a little with carbohydrates but quickly managed to get control of herself again. She had very clearly had less pain and had halved her consumption of pain-relieving tablets. We agreed that she would gradually reduce her intake of thyroxine until her next appointment, which went very well without her having any negative symptoms.

After four months, Kari had reduced her weight by 10 kilograms (1 stone 8) and was as good as pain-free. In the last month she had used just one tablet for the pains, and she had quit thyroxine entirely. The metabolic tests were completely normal without the use of drugs, and her triglycerides were normalised. The C-peptide value had been reduced, even though it hadn't been particularly high at the beginning. The values for Micro-CRP and uric acid were still too high, and therefore we agreed that Kari would have them checked with her GP in the future.

Blood test results before and after diet change.

Blood test	Before	After 4 months	Reference range
C-peptide (pmol/L)	669	459	< 700
Triglycerides (mmol/L)	1.82	0.85	< 1.7
Uric acid (μmol/L)	447	450	155–350
Micro-CRP (mg/L)	>20	>20	< 5
TSH (mU/L)	0.66	1.4 0.	20–4.0
FT$_4$ (pmol/L)	17.5	13.6	9.0–22

Psoriatic arthritis

Psoriatic arthritis is a condition with rheumatic joint inflammation, a form of arthritis which can occur among people with the skin disease psoriasis. Psoriatic arthritis most often comes creeping up with swelling, tenderness and reduced mobility in the joints that are attacked. Perhaps 1 % of the population has psoriasis and 10–40 % of these get psoriatic arthritis. The disease starts most often between the ages of 30–50 years. It is generally agreed that it is the body's immune response which results in inflammation being created in the skin and joints. Psoriatic arthritis is as such an autoimmune disease.

Traditional medical treatment of psoriatic arthritis

Traditionally, the treatment starts with anti-inflammatory drugs. Other pharmaceuticals may be considered if these do not help. Another type of treatment is physiotherapy, light therapy and holidays in warm environs. In exceptional cases there is a need for surgery.

Lotte had psoriatic arthritis and type 2 diabetes

Lotte was 66 years old when she sought me out because she wanted to lose weight. She had gained a lot of weight over the last few years and had not been very active because of arthritis, though she went regularly to exercise sessions for retirees. She had never been a big eater, but was fond of high carb foods, especially bread. Lotte struggled with psoriatic arthritis and high blood pressure for many years, received blood pressure treatment and plenty of pain-relieving tablets because of her arthritis. She had arthritis in her fingers, pelvis and back, and her problems had increased with age. Lotte often felt worn out and tired and assumed that it was due to the arthritis. Her weight was 96 kilograms (15 stone 2) and her BMI was 35.2. Her blood pressure was too high, 160/90 mm Hg, even though she used two blood pressure medications. Lotte desired a rapid weight loss, and we started therefore with a low carb VLCD diet.

At her one-month check-up, she had reduced her weight by 6.7 kilograms (1 stone 1), of which 4.3 kilograms (10 pounds) were fat and the rest water. She had felt good during these weeks and she had more energy. The blood tests she had taken before she started the diet showed that the levels for C-peptide, sugar and ALAT were too high and the profile of the fats unfavourable. Lotte didn't know that she had had diabetes. She wanted me to take a new test of her blood sugar. She was greatly pleased to know that it was completely normal.

We agreed that Lotte would replace one powder meal with a meal consisting of meat or fish and vegetables. After two months she came for a check-up and reported happily that the pain in her joints had been considerably reduced. She could move more, and her energy level was great after having reduced her weight by another 5 kilograms (11 pounds), that is to say a total of 11.7 kilograms (1 stone 12). She gradually switched to a regular low carb diet with more fat, and after six months she had reduced her weight by 14.3 kilograms (2 stone 4) and weighed 81.6 kilograms (12 stone 12). She was able to stop using one of her blood pressure tablets. Her blood pressure had been stable at 135/80 mm Hg. Even though Lotte was very fond of bread, she had no problems cutting it out because she liked the new food and felt good on it. In the time that followed, she indulged herself now and then with high carb foods, and it "punished" her by making her feel bloated, as well as tired and achy in her joints. A check of the blood tests with Lotte's GP showed that her values had normalised, and the relationship between the various cholesterol tests had a lot more favourable because she had got more HDL cholesterol and less LDL cholesterol.

Blood test results before and after diet change.

Blood test	Before	After 6 monts	After 18 months	Reference range
Blood sugar (mmol/L)	7.5	5.7		4–6
C-peptide (pmol/L)	1866	715		< 700
Triglycerides (mmol/L)	2.2	1.1		< 1.7
Total cholesterol (mmol/L)	6.8	7.0	6.6	3.9–7.8
HDL cholesterol (mmol/L)	1.0	1.3	1.4	1.0–2.7
Total/HDL cholesterol	6.8	5.4	4.7	Goal < 4.0
LDL cholesterol (mmol/L)	5.1	5.4	4.6	2–5.3
ALAT (U/L)	50	28		8–46

Gingivitis

Gingivitis is a common condition which affects both the gums and the tooth sockets around the teeth. Bad breath and gums that bleed easily are the first symptoms, and they can be quite troublesome. The main cause of gingivitis is remnants of food on the teeth along the edge of the gum; creating an environment for plaque and tartar, which in turn provide favourable conditions for bacteria. The bacteria lead to inflammation in the area and can also result in cavities in the teeth. If you have inflammation in the tissue nearest the tooth, the tooth socket and the supporting part of the jawbone can become damaged. Over time, the teeth can loosen. Risk factors for gingivitis are poor oral hygiene, a dry mouth (saliva hinders bacteria growth), frequent consumption of meals containing sugar, and smoking. People with diabetes have an increased occurrence of gingivitis because of, among other things, a lot of sugar in the blood and a reduced immune response as a result of considerable fluctuations in blood sugar.

Traditional medical treatment of gingivitis

The usual advice is good oral hygiene with the use of a toothbrush, dental floss, toothpicks or special brushes. The mouth should be cleaned often, and quitting smoking is encouraged. The dentist removes plaque and tartar, and with pronounced changes inflamed tissue is cut away. Antibiotic treatment is also used in serious cases.

Nina's gums bled when she merely moved her tongue along her teeth

Nina was referred to me from her regular doctor for help with losing weight. Both Nina's father and brothers have a typical apple shape with a lot of fat on the belly. Nina had been having problems with her weight since her youth and developed gestational diabetes when she was pregnant the second time. During the pregnancy she was treated with long-acting insulin in the morning and evening and fast-acting insulin four times daily. Despite this treatment, the health care personnel were not pleased with her blood sugar values. She was plagued by itching, had steadily increasing liver values and the foetus was 33 % larger than it should have been. Nina was therefore delivered by a Caesarean section six weeks before her due date.

Nina had long been plagued by migraines, asthma and fibromyalgia. She often had stomach pain and constant constipation. For periods during the last few years, her memory and ability to concentrate were impaired. This worried her, because she was only 40 years old. Nina used drugs for migraine and asthma as needed, and she took metformin daily because she was insulin resistant. She ate a regular European diet and a few sweets when she was at parties.

Her weight was now 93.6 kilograms (14 stone 10), and she was unhappy with her large body. I ordered blood tests, and we agreed on a check-up after six weeks because she was going on vacation and didn't want to change diet before the vacation was over. We agreed that she would cut down heavily on the consumption of foods such as bread, potatoes, rice and fruit after the vacation. As a basic dietary supplement I recommended magnesium, a multivitamin tablet and omega-3 capsules.

At the first check-up, Nina reported that she had gone on a low carb diet for two weeks on the vacation and a ketogenic diet for the last four weeks. After only a couple of days she began to feel better, and she hadn't had a migraine in the last three weeks. Her concentration and memory had become much better, for which she was very happy. Her muscle and joint pain had become much weaker, and her bowels functioned as they should. Then she added that, after two or three days, her gums had stopped bleeding! Nina hadn't told about this problem at the first consultation. She told me that her gums had bled for many years. She bled when she merely moved her tongue along her teeth. She didn't use toothpicks, as it started to bleed immediately. When she was at the dentist, she bled so heavily that the dentist had said that the next time she came for treatment she would need a blood transfusion. It was a joke, of course, but he thought it was difficult to treat her with all the blood in her mouth, so he wanted to send her to a specialist.

Her weight had been reduced by 6.9 kilograms (1 stone 1) during the last six weeks. The blood tests that were taken before the dietary changes showed that she had borderline excessive levels of C-peptide, insufficient levels of vitamin D and SHBG and excessive Micro-CRP. A low SHBG value means too much free and active testosterone in the blood, that is to say a hormonal imbalance. The sun had began to get warm again after winter, so I recommended that she sun-bathe regularly in order to get her level of vitamin D up.

Nina had reduced her weight by 10 kilograms (1 stone 8) but had put on 2–3 kilograms (4–6 pounds) in the course of the summer. It had been difficult to resist potato salad, fresh bread and ice cream at all the garden parties. She had noticed that she craved sweets when she ate more carbohydrates. Her stomach pains also came back, and therefore it wasn't so difficult to go back to her diet. Because of the relapse she felt that she needed regular monitoring for a while.

Her blood tests were completely normal after three months, but since the level of vitamin D was still relatively low, I recommended a supplement. Nina has been to the dentist twice after the dietary change, and on those occasions her gums didn't bleed at all. The dentist wondered what had changed.

Blood test results before and after diet change.

Blood test	Before	After 4 months	Reference range
Micro-CRP (mg/L)	>20	7	< 5
Long-term blood sugar (%)	5.8	-	< 6.1
C-peptide (pmol/L)	674	635	< 700
SHBG (nmol/L)	22	44	23–100
Vitamin D_3 (nmol/L)	26	55	50–150

Sugar and inflammation in the mouth

A series of studies show that patients with diabetes often have various inflammatory conditions in the mouth. This also applies to people who have blood sugar values in the upper normal range. Nina had a long-term blood sugar of 5.8 % before the dietary changes, which is relatively high. Unfortunately, I don't have the value of Nina's long-term blood sugar after three months, because an error was made during the taking of a blood sample. But as you can see in the other blood result tables, the long-term blood sugar decreases when the carbohydrate consumption is reduced.

Sarcoidosis

Sarcoidosis is a chronic inflammation in which small cell lumps, called granulomas, are formed any place in the body. The granulomas occur most often in the lungs and the lymph nodes which lie along the rib cage. The cause of the disease is not known. In Norway, it's believed that 25–35 of every 100,000 people have the disease, and it is more frequent among women than men, and most frequently between 20–40 years of age.

Traditional medical treatment of sarcoidosis

Patients who have symptoms of the disease are usually treated with cortisone for a year and a half or more. There is also alternative pharmaceutical treatment.

Ingrid had sarcoidosis but didn't want cortisone treatment

Ingrid was 30 years old when she came to me because she had heard that in was possible to get better from sarcoidosis by changing diet. In her first pregnancy, she got a lung ailment for which she was admitted to hospital. It was not clear what it was, so she was treated with antibiotics in case of pneumonia and with blood-thinning drugs in case of a blood clot in the lung. After the delivery, large lymph nodes were confirmed in her rib cage, and they steadily became larger. Ingrid was very weak, perspired and slept a lot, had pain in her eyes and muscles, an aggravating dry cough, her breathing was heavy, and her mood fluctuated wildly. She was diagnosed with sarcoidosis. The plan was to start up with cortisone (a synthetic hormone which hinders inflammations) at the hospital, but she was reluctant. The last few years she had also gained weight without understanding why. She ate a lot of bread, cakes and biscuits, which she had always done.

Her blood tests showed that she had a high level of vitamin D (200 nmol/L), resulting from the fact that the granulomas produce this vitamin. I advised her to stay out of the sun and not to take any supplement which contained vitamin D. Ingrid had a relatively high C-peptide (705 pmol/L), which contributed to her having developed sarcoidosis and could explain her weight gain. She had a relatively low level of selenium in her blood, so I advised her to eat two Brazil nuts daily. These nuts are particularly rich in selenium, which is part of an enzyme that functions as an antioxidant. Her BMI was 28. She had also had hair growth in places that are common for men but not for women. This was due to an excess of testosterone, which is common with high insulin production.

I explained to her the connection between insulin and being overweight, moods swings, loss of energy and inflammation and recommended she greatly reduce her consumption of carbohydrates and increase her consumption of meat, fish, poultry, eggs, dairy products without added sugar, nuts and vegetables. She was advised to eat natural, unprocessed food and plenty of oily fish, because it contains omega-3 fatty acids which dampen and counteract inflammations. She went home and pondered over just how important this could be. After a couple of weeks, she threw out all her "garbage food", as she called it, and began to eat natural animal-based foods and a lot of vegetables and nuts.

Four weeks later she returned and reported that she had more energy, much better breathing, less coughing and less pain in her eyes and muscles. Her mood was stable, which her husband particularly liked. Her weight had gone down by 7 kilograms (1 stone), which of course was a bonus.

Ingrid went for a check-up at the hospital as agreed. She was told that her granulomas had become smaller, and she in turn informed the specialists that she had got rid of many of her symptoms. She told them that she had been to see me, and about the changes she had made with her diet. The feedback was that the diet clearly didn't have anything to do with this disease. Ingrid became a little confused over this message. She began to eat bread, cakes and biscuits again, since it couldn't have any significance. After a few days her symptoms increased, her mood sank and gradually she noticed an increasing hair growth.

Ingrid came back to me and I advised her to trust her own body. So she returned to the low carb diet and was again as good as rid of her symptoms. I didn't see her after this but would have liked to follow her up further. In any event, she learnt how important diet is to health.

After two-and-a-half years, I received an e-mail message from Ingrid, in which she said that she was well, and that she hadn't been using cortisone tablets. She had been pregnant during this period, and so she had been extra careful with food and had gained little weight. Towards the end of the pregnancy, some of the symptoms of sarcoidosis had returned, but they disappeared after the delivery.

Due to lactating and little sleep, it was difficult for her to stay away from sweet foods, but she noticed that she just became more tired and worn out afterwards. Some days she had a dry cough, but it came during periods when she ate too much carbohydrate-rich food. Ingrid had noticed that the hormonal system affects the disease, and she thinks that women with sarcoidosis need extra monitoring during periods when they are pregnant and lactating. She feels that she needs more knowledge about the significance of diet for health and therefore wishes a new consultation with me.

ME

What is ME?

ME, or chronic fatigue syndrome, is a term for a disorder which mainly consists of an abnormal feeling of fatigue and lack of energy, that lasts for more than six months. The term ME (myalgic encephalopathy) should actually be avoided, as it suggests that the causal circumstances behind the diagnosis are definitively known – but, in actuality, they are still unclear. The reason that this abbreviation is used so much is probably because it is easier to say ME than chronic fatigue syndrome. I myself use the shortest term. Some think that the disorder primarily has a psychological cause, while others think it has a defined external cause, such as viral infections and/or head injuries, for example. Most agree that it involves a physical disease condition.

In addition to the fatigue itself, the patient must have at least four of the symptoms below for more than six months in order to be diagnosed with ME:

- Impaired memory or concentration
- Sore throat
- Tender lymph nodes on the throat or in the arm pits
- Chronic muscle pain
- Chronic pain from several joints
- Headaches that have not been present previously
- Dizziness

- Unstable blood pressure
- Increased tendency to perspire
- Nausea
- Intestinal problems (diarrhoea, constipation, gas pains)
- Tiredness despite enough sleep and rest
- Feeling of illness after physical activity

Tiredness is a symptom of many disorders, and if you look at the list above, you will perhaps recognise many of the symptoms from the patient case histories I have presented.

It's difficult to estimate the occurrence of ME in the population because it is defined somewhat differently by different doctors, but after an adjustment for other diseases (the symptoms of ME can be confused with the symptoms of other diseases), it seems to be approximately 0.2–0.5 %. The disease occurs more frequently among women (75 % of all cases), and the occurrence is clearly lower among children than among adults. The average age for the appearance of the disease is between 29 and 35 years.

Traditional medical treatment of ME

There is no well-documented treatment of ME. None of the current medications relieve the condition. Some therapists emphasise exercise, others behavioural therapy.

Hege couldn't work because of ME

Hege sought help from me by telephone when she was 39 years old. Five years earlier she had lost all energy and was diagnosed with ME. She went to rehabilitation treatment and had applied for disability benefits because she could no longer be in a job. This had been a big transition, as she liked to work and had previously been very active in martial arts.

She was fond of working out and defined herself as an exercise addict.

Hege had confirmed low metabolism and used thyroxine for this. She slept poorly and woke several times each night, was bothered greatly with hot flushes, which she thought was strange, as she was not of menopause age. The year she was diagnosed, she put on 25 kilograms (3 stone 13), which she disliked greatly. Hege had a constant craving for sweets. Most of the fat she had put on was on her upper body. She didn't feel well, either physically or mentally. She often had attacks of irrational fear, hysterical attacks, had low self-esteem and felt like a loser. This chronic inner anxiety resulted in her body being terribly stressed. Hege told me that she had a large accumulation of fat on her neck (a "buffalo hump"), which can occur with high insulin levels. She was a vegan and ate a lot of grain products, beans, lentils, fruit and vegetables. Her craving for sweets set in at evening time, and then she consumed a lot of fruit, fruit juice, chocolate and ice cream. She still worked out three times a week, even though she often became abnormally worn out after the work-outs.

Her weight was 96 kilograms (15 stone 2) and her BMI 31. I explained to Hege that her great fatigue and craving for sweets were probably caused by fluctuating blood sugar, and that she should consider starting to eat meat and fish to get better. She was willing to consider my proposal, and I looked forward to the next conversation with her. Her blood tests were normal except for an elevated uric acid level. As mentioned earlier, one can have a high level of insulin in the daytime – even though the fasting value isn't particularly high.

Hege requested a new telephone consultation after five

weeks and reported that, in the last few weeks she had consumed just 60 grams of carbohydrates daily. In addition, she had introduced chicken and fish into her diet and thought that it both tasted good and did her good. She had cut out all the sweets in the evening and ate, instead, nuts and cottage cheese. The result was that she felt very well, and the craving for sweets had disappeared entirely. She was finally sleeping at night, she felt more rested and alert and she didn't have hot flushes any longer. Her last menstruation had resulted in less pain and bleeding than she was accustomed to. As a bonus, she had lost her weight. Now she felt mentally strong, her mood was stable, the anxiety and the hysteria attacks had disappeared, she no longer felt like a loser and her body was significantly less stressed. After having reported all these positive effects, she added: "Psychiatric patients would certainly have benefited from such a diet." The symptoms with which Hege had been plagued were caused by fluctuating blood sugar, among other things. Hege felt that she had been given a key to better health and she was highly motivated to continue with this diet. She still becomes worn out after working out, but we are both optimistic and hope that it will soon improve.

Inspired by a magazine, Marianne was cured of ME

This story (slightly edited) demonstrates how patients are seeking new knowledge and are learning from others' experiences.

Hello Sofie Hexeberg,
I found your e-mail address on the Internet. I do hope this e-mail message reaches you. In Hjemmet (a Nor-

wegian weekly magazine for women) number 45/08, there was a report about Mona Farmen who had changed her diet because of, among other things, having diabetes and being overweight. I had the magazine lying around for a long time and had initially ignored the article, because I don't have diabetes myself. But I have been on long-term sick leave because of ME, migraines, muscle pain and two cervical disc prolapses.

I have tried most of the treatment alternatives such as physiotherapy, visiting the chiropractor, homeopathy, rebirthing, etc. Helpful and understanding people gave me hope and courage to continue to become healthy. Even though none of these treatment alternatives helped, it was perhaps a step in the right direction. I had just about given up, because you get little advice from the public health authority and have to feel your way on your own. I have thought about whether it could be something with my diet, but all my blood tests have been fine including allergy tests.

I saw a glimmer of hope when I read that you, as a doctor, would recommend a change in diet (low carb diet) to a series of patients with health problems similar to mine. But I suppose I didn't actually believe entirely that the diet you recommended could help with my problems. That type of diet, I thought, was reserved for patients with type 2 diabetes. Nevertheless, on January 4th 2009, I cut out bread potatoes, rice, pasta, and sugar. My husband was supportive of the diet change, and that was incredibly important for me.

I've worked at a doctor's office (I'm trained as a medical secretary) for a great many years, so I know a little about the scepticism toward this. Now I have the greatest desire to shout about this diet from the rooftops! I recognised quickly that the diet was doing me good, for it felt as though I were waking up from a state of hibernation. I've got my energy back and have much less pain in my head and in my body. Recently I was granted time-limited disability benefits, but I feel that my desire to work has returned, and I actually don't want to stay at home longer, even though I have three children from 7–15 years of age. Four months after the change in diet, I applied for various positions and now work four hours every day in a shop.

I am so grateful for the fact that you came forward in this article and that I read it! I dearly hope that many more people get the chance to do this – changing your diet is not that hard! I feel full all the time and have much more energy and drive. As a bonus, I've reduced my weight by 8 kilograms (1 stone 4).

Thank you! Please convey my thanks to your patient who dared to come forward with her story.

Best regards,
Marianne

ME often occurs in conjunction with other diseases

Patients with ME often have various disorders, such as obesity, diabetes, hypothyroidism, migraines, and muscle and joint pain. My experience is that all such symptoms have a common cause, namely significant blood sugar fluctuations and a high insulin level.

Polycystic ovary syndrome (PCOS)

What is PCOS?

PCOS is a collection of symptoms and findings, of which the most common are:

- Cysts on the ovaries
- Irregular (among 30 % of women) or absence of menstruation (among 50 % of women)
- Blemished, oily skin and pimples
- Hair loss on the head
- Hair growth in places where ordinarily only men have it (among 60 % of women)
- Increased frequency of early miscarriages
- Infertility
- Insulin resistance and obesity
- A significantly increased risk for type 2 diabetes

A PCOS diagnosis requires that at least two of the three following criteria be met:

- Infrequent menstruation or total lack of menstruation over time
- Excess testosterone – hair growth in places which are

natural for men (face, chest, belly, back) and abnormally heavy hair growth on the arms and legs.

- At least one ovary with many cysts confirmed by ultrasound

Many of the symptoms of PCOS can be attributed to insulin and testosterone. Ultrasound tests can confirm cysts on the ovaries, but it is now thought that cysts are not a requirement for making the diagnosis of PCOS. Women who do not have PCOS can also have cysts on their ovaries.

Around 10 % of women are thought to have PCOS, and many don't know that they have it. Heredity influence is an important predisposing factor. About 40 % of sisters and 20 % of mothers of women with PCOS have the syndrome to a varying degree.

PCOS can pop up at any time during reproductive age, but often it occurs late in the teen years. It is thought that PCOS is the most common cause for hormonal disorders among women of fertile age, and the most frequent reason for not getting pregnant because of inadequate ovulation. At least two out of every three women who have PCOS are overweight. Many of them, both of normal weight and those who are overweight, have insulin resistance and, consequently, an increased risk for type 2 diabetes and cardiovascular disease. The fat accumulates first and foremost around the middle. The occurrence of PCOS has strongly increased during the last 20 years, in step with the way our diets and our lifestyles have changed.

Normal ovaries

Women have one ovary on each side of the uterus. The most important function of the ovaries is to release eggs and pro-

The production of gender hormones is controlled by the hypothalamus in the brain.

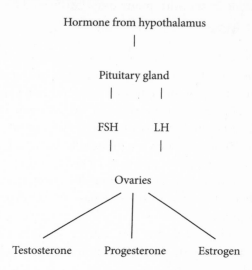

duce the hormones oestrogen (estrogen), testosterone and progesterone. These hormones are regulated by two other hormones that are produced in the pituitary gland in the brain: follicle-stimulating hormone (FSH) and luteinizing hormone (LH). These two hormones influence the development of the follicles and the time of ovulation. The pituitary gland is controlled, in turn, by the hypothalamus which also lies in the brain.

Each egg in the ovaries is surrounded by several layers of cells, and together the egg and these layers are called a follicle. Once a month one of these follicles will grow to approximately two centimetres in diameter and release an egg which enters the Fallopian tube, where a possible fertilisation will occur. A fertilised egg continues to the uterus, where it fastens itself and develops into a foetus. If the woman doesn't become pregnant, the uterine lining is rejected in the form of a menstrual bleeding approximately 14 days after the ovulation.

Polycystic ovaries

Polycystic ovaries either contain many small cysts or one of the ovaries is considerably enlarged. Some of these cysts contain eggs; some are in a resting phase, while others secrete hormones. The cysts are visible on an ultrasonic image.

Causes of PCOS

High LH level: LH is secreted from the pituitary gland in response to signals from the ovaries. With PCOS, the ovaries don't produce sex hormones in the proper proportion. This results in a steady and high secretion of LH to the blood, which leads to an abnormally high production of testosterone. Testosterone inhibits egg maturation, and this results in infrequent and irregular menstruations, blemished skin, masculine hair growth and abdominal obesity.

Obesity, oestrogen and high LH level: Women with PCOS do not have the normal variations in their oestrogen level over the course of a menstrual cycle. They have a constant high level in part, because of formation of oestrogen in fatty tissues. This stimulates increased release of LH from the pituitary gland, which contributes to increased production of testosterone and the formation of cysts in the ovaries.

High insulin level and insulin resistance: The ovaries are relatively sensitive to insulin even if the liver and the muscles are resistant. Insulin has growth hormone properties and leads to the ovaries becoming larger and producing more testosterone than they normally would. In addition, insulin inhibits the production of the transport protein SHBG in the liver, resulting in an increased quantity of free testosterone in the blood. It is the free testosterone (not bound to SHBG) that is biologically active, and in excessive quantities, it can lead to women appearing more masculine.

Traditional medical treatment of PCOS

Weight reduction: It is generally agreed that women with PCOS should reduce their weight where this is an issue. The weight loss should be based on living as healthy a life as possible, including regular exercise, frequent but small meals (4–6 times a day), increased consumption of bread and vegetables and reduced consumption of fat and sweets. If you have PCOS and are overweight and have tried to eat more bread, I suspect that your weight reduction has not been particularly successful.

Medications: Metformin can improve insulin sensitivity and reduce the secretion of sugar from the liver. The medication therefore attacks the problem with the condition. Birth control pills can reduce many of the masculine characteristics, but it takes a long time before an effect on unwanted hair growth is observed.

Desire to become pregnant: In the case of a strong desire to become pregnant, medications are given which promote ovulation. The cells on the ovaries can also be "burnt off" as a step in the treatment of involuntary infertility.

Treatment of embarrassing hair growth: Epilation, electrolysis and laser are methods are used.

My experience with these women is that many don't get treatment at all. Many are quite simply told that some women "are just that way".

Trine had PCOS, hormonal problems and anxiety

Trine came to me when she was 36 years old because she wished to lose weight. The last few years she had put on a lot of weight without entirely understanding why. She ate the same as she had always done and had not changed her exercise habits. She had been diagnosed with PCOS several years previously. She had tried metformin but quit the treatment because it didn't provide any effect worth mentioning, and in addition, she had problems in her gastrointestinal system. Many in her family suffered from obesity, diabetes and heart disease.

Trine ate traditional European food with wholewheat bread, meat, fish, eggs, rice, pasta, potatoes and fruit. She didn't eat a lot of sweets and had tried various slimming diets but didn't think the results were in proportion to the effort. Her weight had crept up to 99 kilograms (15 stone 8) and her BMI was 35.1. She had blemished skin, unwanted hair growth, heavy menstrual bleeding and pain, PMS, fatigue and a lot of fluid in her body. Her blood tests showed excessive levels of C-peptide and uric acid, and the profile of fats in her blood was unfavourable. Her blood sugar was normal; it can be normal over the long term if the pancreas produces enough insulin. Trine had heard about VLCD and wished to try this diet. Some patients think this provides a good start because they break their habits and know exactly what they are to eat at first.

I spoke with Trine on the telephone after three weeks,

and at that time she had reduced her weight by 7 kilograms (1 stone 1). She had acquired a lot more energy and noticed clearly that she had less fluid in her body and that her clothes hung more loosely. At her last menstruation, she had less PMS, bleeding and pain than previously. She was no longer bothered by feeling famished or craving sweets as she used to. Her skin had got much better; she had smaller pores and fewer pimples. These are results I often see in my practice.

The most fantastic thing was that she had got rid of a terrible anxiety that plagued her for many years. She didn't mention this problem at the initial consultation, because she thought it had a natural explanation. She had had a difficult upbringing. The problems were so great that at times she almost didn't dare to go out, sit in a car or look at the news. The fact that this anxiety disappeared when she changed diet indicates that it was contingent on a reactive hypoglycaemia. That means that one gets low blood sugar as a result of excessive insulin production after a high carb meal. When the blood sugar dips, the body produces hormones to get the blood sugar up again. One of these is adrenalin, and a lot of adrenalin results in symptoms such as trembling, sweating, distress, heart palpitations and anxiety.

Trine gradually replaced the VLCD products with meat, fish, eggs, berries, nuts, unsweetened dairy products and low carb bread. She had worked out regularly before, but gradually she introduced more strength training into the sessions. After four months, she had reduced her weight by 17 kilograms (2 stone 9) and felt in top form. The hair growth Trine used to have on her face and on her belly started to go away, and of course she appreciated that greatly. Her weight goal was 70 kilograms (11 stone). She didn't want to take new blood tests, apart from the insulin test, before this goal was reached. She felt that she had been rewarded for her efforts when I told her that her level of C-peptide had been normalised in the course of these four months.

Trine notices that her anxiety symptoms return if she indulges in carbohydrates. Often this also applies to caffeine, which contributes to raising the adrenalin level. Some people can drink eight cups of strong coffee without noticing anything, while others have trembling, sleep problems and anxiety from one or two cups.

Sølvi had PCOS, irregular menstruation and obesity

Sølvi weighed 70 kilograms (11 stone) when she was 18 years old and felt fine at this weight. Gradually her weight began to increase, and the result became an additional 50 kilograms (7 stone 12) in six years without her understanding why. She ate a regular European diet but admitted that she had previously eaten a good deal of chocolate and potato crisps. She didn't, however, eat any more than her friends who were slim. Gradually her craving for sweets increased, but she tried to stay away from sweets because of the weight problem. Since she had menstruated only two times during the past year, (the last time being six months previously), I referred her to a gynaecologist. The examinations showed many cysts on her ovaries, and the blood tests showed that she had insulin resistance and excessive testosterone. She was diagnosed with PCOS and was referred to me to help with her weight reduction and normalising of her hormonal disorder.

Many of Sølvi's relatives struggle with obesity, especially on her father's side. They have a classic apple shape with a large belly and little fat on the backside and hips. Her father's mother has type 2 diabetes and uses blood sugar-reducing medication. The blood tests I had ordered showed that Sølvi's levels of C-peptide (1332 pmol/L), Micro-CRP (15 mg/L) and uric acid (524 μmol/L) were too high, while her levels of SHBG (17 nmol/L) and vitamin D (26 nmol/L) were too low. I recommended a supplement of vitamin D and sunbathing in the summer. Her weight was 113.3 kilograms (17 stone 12), and BMI was 40.6. I advised Sølvi to cut out all sweets and gradually reduce her consumption of starchy foods such as bread, potatoes, rice and pasta.

When she came for a check-up after four weeks, she reported with pleasure that she had menstruated only one week after she started the dietary changes. This result motivated her enormously to continue with the low carb diet. In the course of four weeks, she had also reduced her weight by 5.4 kilograms (12 pounds), of which 4.9 kilograms (11 pounds) was fat. Sølvi hadn't been looking to lose weight but to keep her carbohydrate consumption low in order to achieve hormonal balance. Her new diet gave her a lot more energy so that she had begun to take a three-mile walk daily. As a motivational factor, she used a pedometer, which showed 10–20,000 steps each day.

Her menstruation continued to come once a month, and Sølvi felt like a woman again. Many women think menstruation is a bother, but women with PCOS are grateful every time it comes.

Sugar, insulin and PCOS

Women with PCOS very often have insulin resistance, and approximately 20 percent of overweight women with PCOS have reduced sugar tolerance or diabetes during the ages of 20–30 years. With this there often follows high blood pressure, an unfavourable profile of the fats in the blood, increased inflammation in the body and heart disease. Official dietary advice for women with PCOS is a hich carb/low fat diet. But doesn't that seem a little contradictory when it is actually sugar and insulin which are the cause of the whole problem? It's my opinion that patients with PCOS must be treated with a low carb diet in the same way as other people with insulin resistance. It has a striking effect on obesity, blood sugar, menstruation cycle, skin and hair.

Monika had PCOS, diabetes, hypothyroidism and high blood pressure

Monika was 36 years old when she was referred to me by her gynaecologist. She had many health problems and felt awful. Her weight had started to increase when she was 20 years old, without her having changed anything in her lifestyle. She had always had irregular menstruation – many months often passed between her periods. Ten years before she had been diagnosed with PCOS, and she was plagued with heavy hair growth, especially on her chin, belly, arms and legs. She shaved her face daily, and in the summer she used hours to remove excess body hair. Her gynaecologist had confirmed many cysts in her ovaries, with ultrasound. Her legs were always swollen, her face felt puffy, and her fingers were swollen and stiff. Her stomach was constantly bloated and full of gas. Monika's mood fluctuated a great deal – she could get worked up at the smallest thing, became sad easily and was depressed at times. She had had high blood pressure for two years and had to take four different blood pressure medications. She also had hypothyroidism for five years, and she had used thyroxine just as long. She used birth control pills in order to regulate her menstruation, but they didn't help with all the other problems. No one in Monika's family was affected by obesity, low metabolism or diabetes.

Monika worked out by spinning twice a week in the hope of losing weight. So far, her efforts hadn't had any effect on her fat mass. She started the day with a banana and a bread roll or a fruit yogurt with breakfast cereal. In addition to this she drank a large glass of juice and coffee. For lunch she ate a salad with ham or a bread roll with slices of cheese and meat. Dinner consisted of various types of meat and fish, vegetables and pasta or potatoes. Every day she had three or four pieces of fruit because she had got the message that one must eat five pieces a day. On the weekends she allowed herself a little chocolate or a packet of potato crisps. She wasn't particularly fond of cakes and desserts and therefore seldom ate them.

Christmas was approaching, and Monika was looking forward to a vacation with the family but realised that she couldn't be too radical with her diet during Christmas week itself. We therefore agreed that, for the next check-up, she would greatly reduce her consumption of fruit, bread, pasta and potatoes, but that she could allow herself a little indulgence with the family, who were very fond of food. She didn't wish to weigh herself, because she became so fixated on her weight. I ordered blood tests that she would take before the holiday.

Monika returned after six weeks and, in the preceding four weeks, she had consumed considerably smaller quantities of carbohydrates than previously. She felt that her clothes hung more loosely and that she was retaining less fluid, and her stomach wasn't bloated any longer. She wanted to weigh herself this time, and the scale showed 96.9 kilograms (15 stone 4). We reviewed the blood test results, which showed excessive levels of C-peptide, sugar, triglyc-erides, uric acid, ferritin and gamma GT. Monika wasn't aware that she had diabetes. The metabolic tests were a little unusual, because both TSH and FT_4 were too high. Usually, TSH is low when FT_4 is high (overdosed on thyroxine), or TSH is high when FT_4 is low (an underdose with thyroxine see page 286). She had experienced heart palpitations, a sign that she was getting too much thyroxine. I therefore advised her to reduce the dose. Her blood pressure was normal, so I advised her to quit using the diuretic tablet she used for high blood pressure. She was advised to check her blood pressure after two weeks, and her general practicioner was informed about the change in the treatment with medication.

Monika came for a new check-up after four weeks and reported with a broad smile that she had experienced no further heart palpitations after she had reduced the thyrox-ine dose. Her blood pressure had been normal when checked by the GP. She had noticed that she was retaining less fluid, even though she didn't take a diuretic any longer. Monika felt good and was very motivated to continue with the recommended diet. The carbohydrates she now ate con-sisted of two bread crisps, a piece of fruit, a handful of nuts and lots of vegetables every day. Her weight had gone down by 3.6 kilograms (8 pounds) since the previous visit, and this was so motivating that she was now willing to weigh herself once a month. She was excited to know whether there was any change in her blood tests, so I therefore ordered new tests to be taken before the next check-up.

After another four weeks, she had reduced her weight by another 3.5 kilograms (8 pounds) and she was tremendously pleased. To her great joy, she had noticed that she had a lot less hair on her face and body, and that the hair she still had was softer and brighter than before. Her blood tests were much better, but she was still producing too much insulin. I explained to Monika that her test results would only get better and better as time passed. For some, it takes a little time before C-peptide becomes completely normalised. The thyroxine level in her blood was still too high, and she had experienced a little heart palpitation again. We agreed on reducing the thyroxine dose further. Monika wanted to try to manage on her own, but I advised her to keep seing her regular doctor.

Her GP gradually reduced her other blood pressure medications, and Monika now uses just one of four, while the thyroxine dose has been halved. If she continues with this lifestyle, she will probably be able to quit using the latter tablets as well. She has been for a check-up with her gynaecologist, who found far fewer cysts in her ovaries.

Blood test results before and after diet change.

Blood test	Before	After 3 months	Reference range
Blood sugar (mmol/l)	7.8	6.7	4–6
Long-term blood sugar (%)	7.2	6.1	< 6.1
C-peptide (pmol/L)	1465	1238	< 700
Triglycerides (mmol/L)	3.0	2.3	< 1.7
Ferritin (µg/L)	156	77	13–150
Gamma GT (U/L)	94	41	10–42
Uric acid (µmol/L)	534	410	155–350

Involuntary infertility

What is involuntary infertility?

For couples who decide to have choldren, the likelihood of getting pregnant is about 20 % the first month. For the next 5 months, the likelihood of getting pregnant each month is 20 % for those who remain unpregnant. In the course of one year, approximately 90 % of these women will become pregnant, and after two years approximately 95 %. If a couple is not expecting a child in the course of one year, they are defined as involuntarily infertile. That is to say, approximately 10 % of couples who wish to have a child will have problems in achieving pregnancy. As the years pass, the woman's ability to become pregnant is reduced, and the risk for miscarriages increases. The cause for infertility can lie with the woman, with the man or with both. The most important explanations for involuntary infertility are:

- Disorders in ovulation
- Damage to the Fallopian tubes resulting from infection
- Endometriosis (a condition where the uterine lining is found outside the uterine cavity)
- Reduced sperm quality

Traditional medical treatment
of involuntary infertility

Weight reduction is recommended to those who are over-weight. In other cases, an operation may be considered if the problem involves constricted Fallopian tubes or endometriosis. If the problem is deficient ovulation, the woman receives hormone treatment. Insemination is used to increase the possibility of becoming pregnant. Sperm is then placed in the woman's uterus at the correct moment. Others receive IVF treatment (in vitro fertilisation), which means that the ovum is fertilised outside the woman's body to then be placed in the uterus. About half of those couples classified as "involuntarily infertile" have a child after treatment is completed.

Elna had long wished to become pregnant

Elna had been with the same partner for 15 years and tried to get pregnant for several years without success. She was very sad about this, as all her friends had children and were very busy taking care of them. Elna had long been over-weight, and she had been advised by several different people to lose weight. She was highly motivated and worked out regularly under expert guidance. Despite her efforts over a long period, she didn't lose weight.

Elna told me that both her parents were overweight, and her mother's mother also had type 2 diabetes. Elna was very fond of bread and pasta, which made up a large part of her diet. In addition, she had difficulty staying away from potato crisps, especially on the weekends. Elna was morbidly obese, with a BMI of 47. Not unexpectedly, her blood pressure was high; all of 159/106 mm Hg.

A gynaecological examination showed that everything was normal. Her husband's sperm had been examined and was also found to be normal. Elna wanted to get help for her infertility at the hospital but was informed that they didn't want to help her before she had reached a maximum BMI of 33. Her gynaecologist figured that her infertility was caused by insulin resistance and being overweight, and she was therefore referred to me for further treatment.

Elna wanted a rapid weight reduction because of her intense desire to have a child, and I recommended a low carb diet such as a VLCD. I ordered blood tests and advised her to gradually reduce her carbohydrate consumption before she started with the powder diet.

Elna returned after two weeks. Her blood tests showed that her levels for C-peptide, ferritin and Micro-CRP were too high. In addition, her thyroid gland had begun to fail (elevated TSH), something which is extremely common with obesity and high insulin production. Elna had reduced her carbohydrate consumption as I had suggested, and this had resulted in a weight loss of 1.4 kilograms (3 pounds). She was now very motivated to start with the powder diet, and I explained to her how she should prepare the meals.

At her four-week check-up, Elna had reduced her weight by 7.9 kilograms (1 stone 3), for which she was really pleased. Gradually we replaced the powder meals with foods such as meat, fish, eggs, cheese, crisp bread and a few berries or pieces of fruit. After five months, she had reduced her weight by 20 kilograms (3 stone 2) and her blood tests were normal, except for her Micro-CRP. That is due to the fact that Elna was still carrying too much fat mass, which produces inflammation. Her blood pressure had been reduced to 120/70 mm Hg, which is completely normal. After six months, she became pregnant naturally, and she was overjoyed.

Elna continued to eat low carb food, but I advised her to increase her carbohydrate consumption by approximately five grams per month through the pregnancy. The reason for this was that the foetus also needs a little glucose for, among other things, the growing brain. The pregnant woman can produce the necessary amount of glucose herself, but I see no reason that the body should be burdened with unnecessary work in such a condition. The goal was that she shouldn't gain much weight through the pregnancy. Several studies have shown that this is entirely justifiable on the condition that the food eaten is nutritious. Elna gained a little weight but had an uncomplicated delivery and gave birth to a healthy boy.

Blood test results before and after diet change.

Blood test	Before	After 5 months	Reference range
C-peptide (pmol/L)	920	586	< 700
Micro-CRP (mg/L)	19	20	< 5
Ferritin (µg/L)	172	144	13–150
TSH (mU/L)	5.30	4.47	0.2–4.5

Obesity and reduced fertility

The connection between obesity and reduced fertility is often overlooked. Being overweight reduces fertility significantly and can also cause complications during pregnancy and delivery. A new study has shown that over-weight

women have a different environment in their ovarian follicles than slim women. In obese women, insulin, triglycerides
and CRP are all increased, and SHBG is reduced. This corresponds with findings in the blood of people with insulin
resistance and is a possible explanation for reduced fertility
even among women who have regular menstruation.

Premature menopause

What is premature menopause?

About one percent of all women experience the onset of menopause before they have reached the age of 40. This means that they can no longer have children, and that the body's aging process starts earlier. Women are born with a certain number of immature ova in their ovaries. With cooperation between the brain and the ovaries, a certain number of ova are used each month. Under ordinary circumstances, this results in ovulation and menstruation. However, a hormonal failure can occur in the ovaries, the cause of which can either be that the number of immature ova is reduced, or that the ovaries are not functioning normally.

The reason for these problems is most often unknown, but in approximately one-third of cases the symptoms can be related to another disease. The symptoms for premature menopause are the same as for menopause. They just occur earlier than expected: hot flushes, night sweats, mood swings, fatigue, reduced sexual desire, dry mucous membranes and urinary disorders. A conclusive diagnosis is made by confirming hormonal changes in the blood. These women can also have other hormonal disorders in the adrenal glands, pituitary gland, thyroid gland and pancreas, and they have an increased frequency of autoimmune diseases.

The most important consequences in the long term are an increased risk of cardiovascular disease and osteoporosis.

Traditional medical treatment of premature menopause

There are no medications which can restore ovarian function. Common recommendations are a healthy, low fat diet, exercise, a healthy lifestyle and taking enough calcium and vitamin D. Many doctors also recommend oestrogen replacement, at lest until a more normal age for menopause.

Berit became menopausal at age 38

Berit was referred to a gynaecologist because she had not menstruated for six months, and she was not pregnant. During this period, she had generally felt unwell and had put on 12 kilograms (1 stone 13) in a short time without having changed her lifestyle. Occasionally she got an extreme craving for sweets. She was plagued with hot flushes, was irritated and completely lacked energy. Berit had also noticed that she was retaining more fluid; she felt bloated in her face and swollen in her fingers, calves and ankles. She constantly forgot things she knew how to do, she muddled her words, and her concentration was poor. She got infections easily and had, among other things, pneumonia, which was being treated with antibiotics. She couldn't manage to perform the job she loved and was therefore on sick leave. Even though her metabolic tests had been normal, she had received thyroxine. She had also received diuretic tablets because of the increasing amount of fluid in her body. This hadn't helped with any of her problems. Her gynaecologist confirmed premature menopause with blood tests and referred her to me for dietary advice and weight reduction. Berit weighed 109 kilograms (17 stone 2), her BMI was 33.2 and her blood pressure normal, that is to say 120/80 mm Hg.

I explained to Berit that her problems, in all likelihood, were due to insulin resistance. I explained that, if the cells are resistant to insulin, the pancreas must produce more insulin in order to keep the blood sugar under control. This leads, in turn, to problems with the sex hormones. I advised her to gradually reduce her carbohydrate consumption over the course of a few days and then to consume only 20 grams per day. She was willing to try this if there was hope that she could become healthy again.

Berit came for a check-up after four weeks and reported that she had already felt better after a couple of days on the new diet. Her craving for sweets disappeared, and her energy, concentration and memory became much better. In addition, she had reduced her weight by 6 kilograms (13 pounds), of which 5 kilograms (11 pounds) were fat and 1 kilogram (2 pounds) was water. She noticed clearly that she had less fluid in her body and her face had regained its normal shape.

The blood tests confirmed my suspicion about insulin resistance. The values for C-peptide (1199 pmol/L) and uric acid (512 μmol/L) were too high, and her fasting blood sugar (5.9 mmol/L) was also borderline. Berit was producing a lot of insulin, which is the body's reaction for controlling blood sugar, but now it was unable to maintain strict control of her blood sugar. Berit's metabolic tests were normal, and we agreed that she would gradually reduce her dosage of thyroxine.

Five weeks after she changed diet, she had an ordinary period and was overjoyed. From then on she had a period regularly every fourth week. After six weeks she started working full time again and felt that she had got her life back. Berit started walking several times a week and had energy for family and friends again. A bonus with the dietary change was that her bowel functioned as it should. Berit had suffered from constipation since she was a child, and nothing had even begun to improve the condition. Before the dietary change she would go to the bathroom only twice a week, but on the low carb diet she had a bowel movement every day.

Berit will be monitored further by her regular doctor.

Migraine

What is migraine?

A migraine is a one-sided, pulsing headache which, untreated, can persist for up to three days. The condition generally appears first in puberty. Around 9 % of all women and 3 % of all men are affected. Nearly 20 % of the population experiences one or more migraine attacks in the course of their lives. The condition is most frequent among women in their 40s.

A migraine attack is divided into four phases:

1. The pro-dromal phase can start a day before the headache itself comes. Sensory perceptions change slightly in this phase.
2. Only one of five migraine patients has the aura phase. This phase lasts for up to an hour. In this phase, it is common to have flickering light that flashes across the field of vision, and parts of the visual field may disappear. Some get a tingling and pricking in the hands, and some become dizzy and unsteady.
3. The headache phase is often pulsing, intense and one-sided. Nausea and retching are usual, and intense light and loud sounds are less tolerated.
4. The post-dromal phase is the repercussions after the headache. Sufferers are often worn out and have aching muscles.

The cause of migraines is not known in detail, but there are almost certainly hereditary predispositions. In addition, a range of factors can trigger an attack – for example, stress, red wine, cheese, oranges and chocolate, lack of sleep, irregular meals and menstruation. It is known that, during the migraine attack, a constriction and then a considerable expansion of the arteries in the head occurs.

Traditional medical treatment of migraine

Migraine is traditionally treated with pain-killing medication.

Karita was on sick leave because of migraine and many other health problems

Karita sought help from me when she was 57 years old. She had many physical problems, but what concerned her most was that she constantly felt faint and had to sit down. Simultaneously, her head felt empty, and her memory disappeared. Her mood had also been extremely variable, and at times she was noticeably irritable and angry. She had also noticed a great craving for sweets, so she ate a lot of fruit because she had learnt that it was healthy and good for the body.

Karita tried to stay away from sweets and cakes but was very fond of bread and potatoes, of which she consumed a lot. Many members of Karita's family were overweight, and she too was overweight. She went on walks regularly and worked out in a gym. However, she was plagued with muscle and joint pain which constantly moved to new places. Her knee joints were particularly painful. Magnetic resonance images showed pronounced arthrosis in her knees, and the rheumatologist had said that she had to be monitored with annual check-ups. She itched and became tight in her throat when she ate eggs, paprika, nuts, and pepper and when there was perfume in the air. In addition, she got an upset stomach when she ate egg, so she tried to avoid it.

Karita also had migraines often, which first developed when she was around 30 years old. She had several attacks a month and had to take medication, even though she often became ill or experienced little effect. She noticed clearly when the attacks were coming. On those occasions, she had to arrange relief for her job for the next three days. During the attacks, she had pain in her head and neck and was sick in her entire body. She was nauseous, couldn't manage food and had to lie in bed in the dark with lots of woollen blankets.

In addition to traditional medical treatment, she had tried many alternative treatments. She had cut out various foods, taken supplements of vitamins and minerals and tried an ordered lifestyle. None of this helped. Karita was on sick leave because she couldn't maintain a full time job. The last few years she had greatly reduced her consumption of sweets because she had gotten her diagnosis of insulin resistance confirmed some years earlier. Karita had steadily gained weight, but her blood pressure had always been normal.

When Karita came to me, I explained to her how blood sugar fluctuations and high insulin production could result in many of the symptoms she had. She nodded in recognition – she had a feeling that it had to do with the blood sugar. I told her how low blood sugar leads to increased adrenalin production and, consequently, migraines, and this she also nodded in recognition of. She told me that she had been in hospital twice because of serious allergic reactions, and both times she had received an adrenaline injection. She remembered this very well because she had never had such an intense migraine attack either before or since.

We agreed that she would focus on achieving stable blood sugar levels and not on weight reduction. I advised her to gradually reduce her carbohydrate consumption so that, after a couple of weeks, she only consumed approximately 20 grams per day. She thought it was strange that she should quit using the milk that she was so fond of, but I told her that there are 25 grams of milk sugar in a pint of milk. I also recommended that she take up to 600 milligrams of magnesium every day. This usually has good effect on migraines in combination with a low carb diet.

Four weeks later, she came for a check-up, and we looked at the blood test results together. Her C-peptide value (700 pmol/L) was in the boundary range, and her level of uric acid (493 µmol/L) was too high. She was pleased with the test results because the level of C-peptide had been much higher some years earlier. She had changed to a ketogenic diet and had noticed, during the last few weeks, that her mood had become better and that the migraine attacks were weaker and came more seldom. The pain and the stiffness in her body were getting better, and she felt that she had more energy than before.

One month later, she reported, beaming with joy, that she hadn't had a migraine since her last appointment. The month after, she reported that the pain in her knees was much weaker, and she had not yet had another migraine.

Two months passed before I saw her again, and during this period she had learnt something useful from experience. She had participated in a three-day-long celebration of a 60th birthday, and during this time she had eaten some slices of bread, cakes, and potatoes. Because of these "indul-gences," she again became stiff in her body, and experienced pain in her muscles and joints once again. After the three days, she had gone back to a ketogenic diet, and her body became pain-free. She had eventually discovered that she now tolerated eggs, paprika, nuts, pepper and perfume.

Karita is gradually losing weight and always has magne-sium in her bag. If she feels as if she might develop a head-ache, she takes 500 milligrams of magnesium, and then the headache never materialises. She feels relieved at being migraine-free and, not least, having to worry about approaching attacks. Karita has also taught herself that cheating with carbohydrates carries its own punishment.

When she had been on a low carb diet for six months, she visited the rheumatologist for a new check-up on her knees. The rheumatologist wondered whether anyone had cleaned up inside her knees, for the MRI images were much better than the previous time. The first image show-ed cartilage changes and inflammatory changes, but the striking thing about image number two was that the inflammatory changes were completely gone. She told the rheumatologist that she had been to see me, had eaten a low carb diet for six months and was pain-free. The rheumatologist was surprised but said that perhaps there was something to this thing with diet after all.

Sugar, insulin and migraine

High levels of insulin and reduced sensitivity to insulin have been documented in people who suffer from migraines. Studies have also shown that the catecholamine level in the blood is far higher three hours before a migraine attack than among people who do not have a migraine. Catecholamines are a group of hormones which, among other things, cause the blood vessels to constrict. Adrenalin, noradrenalin and dopamine are all catecholamines. They are produced in the adrenal glands, and production increases when, for example, the person suffers stress and heavy exertion. I have previously written about low blood sugar, and you may remember that the symptoms are unease, trembling, sweating, and heart palpitations. This is due to an increased production of adrenalin, which is the body's response to low blood sugar. Adrenalin, therefore, is one of the hormones which can get the blood sugar up again. Too much adrenalin, however, leads to the constriction of blood vessels and can therefore start a migraine attack. For that reason, a stable blood sugar is extremely important for people who are plagued by migraines.

Magnesium often has a good effect on migraines because it causes the blood vessels to relax. Several studies have shown that magnesium works both preventively and it can alleviate migraine attacks.

Tonje tried medication first for migraine

Tonje had been plagued with migraines since her teenage years, and whenever she had an attack, she would be completely worn out and she couldn't go to work. She had tried various blood pressure medication for the migraines, but the side-effects were greater than the improvement she got from them. A specialist had prescribed some other medicines which worked quite well. On these drugs she had attacks only a few days every week. She had a prolapse in her neck for which she was receiving treatment from a chiropractor, since a prolapse can also give head pain.

Tonje had been overweight since she was a teenager, and she had been troubled by an upset stomach for as long as she could remember. Blood tests and intestinal examinations had shown an intolerance to the proteins in cows' milk and grain (casein and gluten). She got diarrhoea if she drank milk and became bloated and got stomach pain when she ate bread. Many members of her family were obese, and both her mother's father and an uncle had type 2 diabetes.

Tonje came to me because she had heard that blood sugar could be responsible for her migraines, and she wished to do whatever she could to avoid being dependent on the drugs she now used. She also wanted to lose weight because she was starting to become afraid of the health consequences of being overweight. She was a typical yo-yo dieter who had tried a wide range of diets. At times, she ate for comfort because she felt that nothing worked. Tonje had already been referred for breast reduction because she had such pain in her shoulders from her heavy breasts, and because this could alleviate her neck pain. Before the operation, she had to quit using migraine medication, which resulted in her getting a headache every day. Tonje weighed 101.4 kilograms (15 stone 14). I explained carefully to her the connection between food, blood sugar, insulin, obesity and migraine. We agreed that she would stop eating sweets and take 200 milligrams of magnesium twice daily.

After a month she returned, having had the breast reduction operation. She had limited her consumption of carbohydrates and had lost 4.3 kilograms (10 pounds) of weight, of which 600 grams (1.3 pounds) was the breast tissue that was removed. She had suffered from a constant headache for the first ten days after the operation and had, therefore, started taking medication for her migraines again. Her blood tests showed an excessive level of C-peptide and an unfavourable profile of fats in the blood. We agreed that she would eat even fewer carbohydrates, so that she would only consume approximately 20 grams per day. I also advised her to increase her consumption of natural fat.

After another four weeks, Tonje came for a check-up and reported that she hadn't managed to eat as few carbohydrates as I had recommended. Nevertheless, she felt that she was on a good path with the new diet, and her weight had gone down by a further 2.8 kilograms (6 pounds).

At the next check-up, Tonje had reduced her weight by another 4.2 kilograms (9 pounds) – that is to say, a total of 11.3 kilograms (1 stone 11) – and all her blood tests were normal. She reported, with great pleasure, that her husband had begun the same diet, and he had lost 8 kilograms (1 stone 4) in six weeks. She was happy for him, but thought it was a little unfair that he was losing weight so much faster than her! I told Tonje that this often happens, partly because men have greater muscle mass than women. She continued with the weight reduction and was 15 kilograms (2 stone 5) lighter after four months. At that time, she was as good as rid of the migraine attacks. She now took no regular medication, but on occasion she had to take a tablet for a migraine right before menstruation. Tonje wants to lose even more weight and is aware that she needs regular monitoring to keep up her motivation.

Blood test results before and after diet change.

Blood test	Before	After 3 months	Reference range
C-peptide (pmol/L)	962	641	< 700
Triglycerides (mmol/L)	2.96	1.27	< 1.7
Total cholesterol (mmol/L)	6.9	6.4	3.3–6.9
HDL cholesterol (mmol/L)	1.2	1.6	1.0–2.7
Total/HDL cholesterol	5.8	4.0	<4
LDL cholesterol (mmol/L)	4.6	4.2	1.4–4.7

Preventive measures for migraine

- Have a structured lifestyle.
- Avoid stressful situations as far as possible.
- Get enough sleep.
- Eat low carb food to maintain stable blood sugar levels.
- Avoid food and beverages which from experience trigger attacks – cheese, oranges, chocolate and red wine are the classic "dangers" which you can try to eliminate first.
- Eat a lot of seeds and nuts in order to get plenty of magnesium.
- Take up to 600 mg of magnesium in tablet form daily divided into two doses – talk with your doctor about this if you have a chronic disease.

Atrial fibrillation

What is atrial fibrillation?

The heart has an electric conduction system, and electrical impulses are released from the right atrium. These spread out into the heart to the left atrium and then on to both the heart chambers. The electrical impulses set off the contractions that cause the blood that is inside the heart to be pumped out in the body's blood vessels. With atrial fibrillation, the electrical impulses are released much faster than what is normal. The result is that the heart's pumping becomes less efficient. Atrial fibrillation is rare before the age of 60 but occurs among 6–8 % of people in their 70s and among 10 % of all 80 year olds.

The most common causes of atrial fibrillation is another heart disease, high metabolism, alcoholism and chronic lung disease. The symptoms of atrial fibrillation are strong and irregular heart palpitations, which often means that the sufferer quickly becomes worn out and out of breath. The diagnosis is often made by feeling an extremely irregular pulse. An ECG (electrocardiogram) is necessary, however, to make a reliable diagnosis.

Differentiation of atrial fibrillation

Paroxysmal atrial fibrillation: Episodes of atrial fibrillation that stop on their own. Over time it often becomes permanent.

Persistent atrial fibrillation: Atrial fibrillation which doesn't stop on its own but which may stop with the aid of medication or electroshock to the heart. Over time it often becomes permanent.

Permanent atrial fibrillation: Constant atrial fibrillation which does not disappear with the aid of treatment.

Traditional medical treatment of atrial fibrillation

The goal is to reduce the symptoms and lessen the burden on the heart:

- With newly developed atrial fibrillation, one usually attempts to get a normal heart rhythm back with the aid of medication.
- If medication is not successful, electroshock to the heart can, in many cases, give the heart the proper rhythm.
- Ablation therapy is a new method for treatment of paroxysmal atrial fibrillation – electrodes are put into the heart through a blood vessel in order to localise the abnormal electrical pathways, which then are destroyed.
- Because of the risk of blood clots, blood-thinning treatment is recommended with permanent or frequent paroxysmal atrial fibrillation.
- In the case of permanent atrial fibrillation, medication that lowers the heart rhythm is often used.

Øyvind was to be operated on for atrial fibrillation

Øyvind was 45 years old when he sought me out. He had been healthy for most of his life, except that he sometimes had migraines. During the previous year he had experienced atrial fibrillation many times and had been referred for ablation at the hospital.

The first time he had an attack, he managed to control it by simply relaxing with his wife and drinking a few glasses of wine. He had read that coffee wasn't good for him, so he switched to decaffeinated coffee. Øyvind also understood that stress could trigger atrial fibrillation, so he tried to organise his days with the least possible stress. He drank moderate amounts of alcohol and didn't smoke, but the atrial fibrillation reoccured many times.

The first time Øyvind came to the hospital to receive treatment, he changed to a normal rhythm while the nurse was putting a needle in the vessel in his hand. On several occasions he received medication directly into the blood, which reinstated a normal rhythm. The fourth time he came to the hospital, medication didn't help, and he had to be sedated and have electroshock. He underwent this treatment several times, until the doctors at the hospital decided that he had to go to a university hospital to have an ablation performed.

Øyvind dreaded the surgical procedure and came to me to hear whether there was something he could do with his diet that could improve his condition. Øyvind ate whole-wheat bread for breakfast and lunch, dinner with potatoes, rice and pasta and usually a sandwich in the evening. He was slim, and his blood tests were completely normal. I explained to Øyvind that a lot of adrenalin can trigger atrial fibrillation. If he ate fewer carbohydrates, he would avoid large fluctuations in his blood sugar and, consequently, he would have a lower adrenalin level. He was willing to try this, and we agreed that, in the course of a week, he would cut down to approximately 50 grams of carbohydrates per day divided among his meals. I explained to him what he was to eat and gave him plenty of written information, including some simple recipes. He was happy when I gave him a bread recipe, for he didn't understand how he would manage without bread. Øyvind was somewhat interested in dietary supplements, and he took a multivitamin tablet and two capsules of cod liver oil daily. I also recommended 600 milligrams of magnesium per day, and a zinc supplement because he had a bad taste in his mouth and his gums bled constantly.

Øyvind returned after four weeks and reported that his general condition had become much better over the course of these weeks. He wasn't as hungry any longer, and the bloated feeling in his stomach had disappeared. In addition, he had acquired more energy and slept better than before. His mood was also more stable, and his gums had complet-ely stopped bleeding when he cleaned his teeth. His wife was extremely pleased because the bad breath was gone. Best of all, he hadn't had a migraine in four weeks. Nor did he expe-rience any atrial fibrillation – but it was too early to tell whether it would last.

I have had regular contact with Øyvind the last few years, and he has reported that he has had neither atrial fibrillation nor migraines since he changed his diet and started with magnesium three years ago. He had felt that he was about to get a migraine attack in some stressful situations, but he had countered it with an extra dose of magnesium.

Sugar, insulin and atrial fibrillation

As explained earlier, a high consumption of carbohydrates can lead to a rapid decline in blood sugar. That's due to the fact that a lot of sugar in the blood triggers a lot of insulin, which in turn leads to the sugar being absorbed in the cells. The rapid decline in blood sugar can, in turn, trigger an increased secretion of glucagon, cortisol and adrenalin, three hormones which contribute to blood sugar increasing. Adrenalin stimulates the heart, but if the heart becomes over-stimulated, adrenalin can contribute to atrial fibrillation being triggered. Cortisol is known to be, among other things, a stress hormone, and stress can trigger atrial fibrillation. It has been shown that the cortisol level in the blood increases when the insulin level increases. In other words, when you consume a lot of carbohydrates, you get increased secretion of two hormones, both of which contribute to electrical disorders in the heart. It has also been shown that the consumption of a lot of carbohydrates over a long period reduces the body's stores of magnesium and consequently increases the body's need for magnesium.

We have approximately 25 grams of magnesium in the body, and half of this is located in the skeleton. Magnesium is a cofactor in over 300 enzymes in the body and is necessary for the normal function of the heart, muscles and the body's metabolism. Normally the heart has a high magnesium content, and this mineral contributes to maintaining the electrical potential across the cell membranes in nerve and muscle cells. This is critical for everything functioning as it should.

The following can lead to magnesium deficiency:

- Unbalanced diet
- Vitamin D deficiency
- Too much bran in the diet
- Large consumption of milk products and calcium
- Large consumption of coffee
- High alcohol consumption
- High consumption of carbohydrates
- High insulin level
- Diabetes
- Kidney disease
- Chronic diarrhoea
- High metabolism
- Deficient uptake of nutrients in the intestine
- Stress
- Heavy sweating
- Weight-loss diets
- Ageing
- Pregnancy
- Some pharmaceuticals, especially diuretics

Foods which contain a lot of magnesium.

Food	mg/100g
Pumpkin seeds, Squash seeds	535
Brazil nuts	410
Sunflower seeds	354
Sesame seeds	350
Almonds, Cashews	270
Peanuts	210
Monkfish	190
Flax seeds, crushed	180
Walnuts, Hazel nuts	160

As the table above shows, you will get plenty of magnesium by including nuts and seeds in your diet. Authorities recommend a daily intake of 280 milligrams for women (including lactating and pregnant women) and 350 milligrams for men. For children, the requirement is stipulated at 120–280 milligrams depending on the age og the child.

The amount we have in the body is determined, not just by the intake but also by the uptake, consumption and excretion. A blood test shows how much magnesium there is in the blood but says nothing about whether there is enough in the cells. In order to find out, we must examine how much magnesium there is in the blood cells or analyse the excretion in the urine. Many nutritional experts think that the need for magnesium is greater than official recommendations and that it varies from individual to individual.

The low carb diet as medication

If you want to lose weight

If you eat few carbohydrates, you reduce your body's need for insulin and more easily burn the fat you eat – as well as the body's own fat. Low carb diets are controversial, despite the fact that their effects have been known ever since Jean-Anthelme Brillat-Savarin described them in 1825. Today there are a number of newer studies which show the advantages of a reduced consumption of carbohydrates for patients with, for example, obesity, types 1 and 2 diabetes and epilepsy. Earlier in the book I have described the negative consequences of high carbohydrate consumption and insulin levels. For that reason, my dietary recommendation will always include eating a low carb diet.

The diet for you

We have different food preferences, different psyches and goals, and we are in different phases of life. A weight reduction program or a maintenance diet that works well for your friend may, therefore, be completely wrong for you. It's important that your particular diet suits your social situation and psyche and your health problems or diseases.

Perhaps you wish to get rid of some extra weight rapidly, or perhaps you want to take more time. The usual treatment for overweight is a low fat, high carb, low calorie diet and exercise. This can cure obesity and overweight for some people, but there are many others for whom it doesn't work. Based on my own and others' clinical experience, I believe that the most important thing is to manage a low carb diet which you can live with over time. If the diet is too strict, you won't be able to maintain it, and the result is yet another unsuccessful diet. It's therefore important to think through which carbohydrates are especially important to you – and simultaneously be clear that you cannot eat masses of carbohydrates every day all week long. One day a piece of fruit can be a little extra treat, another day a slice of wholewheat bread, a little pasta or a small potato. You have to negotiate with yourself a little. That way you don't need to abstain from all the foods you are accustomed to eating. Some people have a real problem eating bacon. You can't coerce people to eat bacon and eggs for breakfast if it troubles their conscience and they think it will make them gain weight. A ham omelette is often more acceptable, so many begin there. The definition of a low carb diet varies, but the common denominator is a low consumption of carbohydrates. As a member of the board of directors of Foreningen kostreform ved overvekt og sukkersykdommer (The Society for Dietary Reform on Overweight and Sugar Diseases) and a practising physician, I recommend a diet which research and experience have shown can cure various diseases, provide effective weight loss and results in diabetics being able to manage without (or with less) insulin and other medication. This often means a diet restricted to as few as 20–30 grams of carbohydrates per day to begin with, and a maximum of 80–100 after the dieter is rid of his or her health problems.

Diets restricted to 50–70 gram carbohydrates per day

Foods such as meat, fish, shellfish, poultry, eggs, cheese, butter and oils contain very few or no carbohydrates. You can therefore eat these in the amounts that make you comfortably full. The carbohydrate sources should primarily be of a type that gives the lowest possible blood sugar increase. For instance: vegetables, nuts, seeds, berries, milk products without added sugar, pulses, whole grains and fruit. The most important thing is, however, to limit the amount of carbohydrates in your diet. In the following table you can see some examples of how many carbohydrates there are in specified portions of various foods. The values are approximate. When you shop, I recommend that you read the declarations to find out how many carbohydrates products contain. You can also look up the amount of carbohydrates by using the summary at the back of this book.

The amount of carbohydrates (CH)
in specified portions of some common food products.
The numbers have been rounded off.

Food product	Portion	Grams CH in specified portion	Grams CH in 100 gram
Bread products			
Protein bread	1 slice, 20 g	2	10
Rye crisp	1 piece	6	66
White bread	1 slice, 35 g	12	47
Whole grain rye bread	1 slice, 35 g	14	39
Roll, wholewheat	1 piece, 50 g	26	52
Wheat tortilla	1 piece, large	28	48

Breakfast cereal			
Muesli	30 g	7	24
All-Bran Plus	30 g	14	47
Rolled oats	30 g	19	63
Cornflakes	30 g	24	82
Milk and milk products			
Whipping cream	1 dl (4 oz)	3 (4)	3 (4)
Natural yogurt	100 g	6	6
Milk	2 dl (8 oz)	9 (11)	5 (6)
Fruit yogurt	150 g	18	12
Vegetables, beans and potatoes			
Tomato	1 piece, 60 g	1.5	2.5
Iceberg lettuce	200 g	3	1.5
Broccoli	200 g	4	2
Carrot	1 piece, 70 g	5	7
Boiled potato	1 piece 150 g	26	17
Beans in tomato sauce	150 g	21	14
French Fries	150 g	60	40
Berries and fruit			
Raspberries	150 g	5	3
Strawberries	150 g	10	7
Blueberries	150 g	11	8
Orange without peel	1 piece, 150 g	11	7
Apple	1 piece, 150 g	16	10
Green Grapes	150 g	24	16
Banana	1 piece, 150 g	27	18
Nuts, almonds and snacks			
Bacon rinds	50	0.1	0.2
Walnuts	50	1.5	3

Almonds	50	3.5	7
Peanuts	50	6	13
Potato crisps, low fat	50	31	63
Rice, pasta and pizza			
Brown rice, boiled	80 g	16	20
White rice, boiled	80 g	21	26
Spaghetti, boiled	80 g	21	27
Waffles, cakes and chocolate			
Waffle	1 piece, 20 g	5	25
Chocolate 70 %	50 g	15	30
Chocolate cake with icing	1 piece, 40 g	19	47
Wheat bun without raisins	1 piece, 50 g	27	55
Milk chocolate	50 g	27	53
Pick 'n' Mix without chocolate	50 g	44	89
Juice, fruit drinks and soft drinks			
Orange juice	150 ml (5 oz.)	15	10
Mixed berry juice with water	150 ml (5 oz.)	15	10
Soft drink	500 ml (16 oz.)	50	10

Here's how you reduce your carbohydrate consumption

Many people today consume large amounts of carbohydrates from eating starchy foods, fruit, sweet dairy products, soft drinks and sweets. Moving directly from this to a low carbohydrate diet, may give you withdrawal symptoms such as headaches, dizziness, mood swings, depression, irritability and fatigue. In order to avoid this, it's important that you use one or two weeks to gradually reduce your carbohydrate consumption. A low carb diet consisting of the fewest possible processed foods will ensure a stable and relatively low blood sugar level, good metabolism, plenty of vitamins, minerals and anti-oxidants, maintenance of muscle mass, a sense of being full, hormonal balance and a good immune response. In this gradual reduction phase, you needn't focus on the amount of food or that you're supposed to lose weight.

Mealtimes

Most people find it natural to eat breakfast, lunch and dinner, while others prefer breakfast, dinner and supper. The choice is yours. Regardless, you should take time with your food and chew it well. The feeling of being full will first appear actually 20–30 minutes after you started to eat. If you eat quickly, you'll take in more food than necessary. Eat until you are comfortably full, not completely gorged.

There's no law of nature that says that we have to eat breakfast. But if you skip breakfast, it often results in you eating too much in the evening and being less critical of what you're eating. In other words, most people benefit from eating breakfast. In the course of the day, you don't need to eat when you're not hungry or don't feel a physical need for food. It's not necessary to eat many snacks when you eat a high fat/low carb diet and have stable blood sugar. At times in between meals, you can draw on your own fat stores from the belly, thighs and other areas. If you like eating small portions best, you may, of course, need a little extra food in between your main meals.

Ten Top tips for the person who wants to eat fewer carbohydrates and have stable blood sugar levels

1. Cut out soft drinks and other sweet beverages and avoid large amounts of milk – drink water instead, water with lemon, or mineral water.

2. Cut out sugar, cakes, buns, sweet chocolate, candy and the like – ordinary sugar can be replaced with erythritol or other sweeteners that don't elevate your blood sugar levels.

3. Reduce your consumption of starchy foods such as bread, potatoes, rice and pasta.

4. Eat fruit instead of drinking juice – 1 litre of orange juice contains about 100 grams of sugar.

5. Avoid diet soft drinks – many people get a craving for something really sweet when they drink diet soft drinks. It's important that you wean yourself from constantly having to have something sweet in your mouth.

6. Eat a maximum of one piece of fruit per day. Choose instead more berries and vegetables.

7. Use products such as natural yogurt, natural cultured milk, cottage cheese, sour cream, crème fraîche and whipping cream in food if you tolerate it. Most people tolerate prepared milk products better than sweet milk.

8. Increase your consumption of natural fat and proteins. This makes you feel full longer and reduces the need for carbohydrates.

9. Always have some foods available to satisfy a sudden hungry feeling when you are overworked, tired or stressed – nuts, cheese, cured meat, a few berries with cream, a protein bar or some bits of 70–85 % dark chocolate.

10. Try supplements of chromium and/or magnesium and increase your fat consumption if you're constantly "longing" for carbohydrates.

Breakfast

Breakfast is the meal of the day that ought to contain the most fat and proteins and the fewest carbohydrates. Eating a lot of fat provides a good feeling of fullness which results in you needing smaller portions and not needing to eat as often as before. By eating few carbohydrates, you maintain the fat metabolism which started during the night. Here are some tips for approaching this goal:

- *Bread*: Cut thinner slices of bread and reduce the number of slices of bread you eat. Use coarser breads such as pumpernickel, whole grain rye bread recipe, coarse Danish rye bread or low carb bread. Eat protein-rich spreads, such as shrimp, smoked salmon, hot-smoked mackerel, sardines, herring, mackerel in tomato sauce, 100 % meat spreads, eggs, cheese or cottage cheese.
- *Porridge:* Make the porridge from rolled oats and water or milk. Mix in cottage cheese, cream or sour cream and chopped nuts, almonds or seeds and sprinkle on some fresh berries. Enjoy it with erythritol and cinnamon.
- *Muesli*: Make your own muesli with fewer carbohydrates than those that are found in the shops. Use equal parts of multi-grain cereal, rolled oats, soya flakes and plenty of almonds, nuts and seeds. Add berries and/or erythritol if you want a sweeter taste and natural yogurt or coconut milk.
- *Smoothie*: Make a smoothie of berries or fruit and natural yogurt, natural cultured milk, whipping cream or coco-

nut milk, eggs and nuts or seeds. See what you like. The smoothie can be sweetened as desired with erythritol.

- **Eggs**: Make an omelette with chopped vegetables and ham, cheese and cream. Have fried eggs and bacon, make scrambled eggs and add smoked salmon, used hard-boiled eggs and avocado or make a low carb pancake (page 254). You can add a few cut-up vegetables to the egg dishes and some berries or grated apple to the pancake. These dishes contain few carbohydrates, provide a good start to the day and keep you full for a long time.

Lunch

- **Salad**: Choose different vegetables and vary them with chicken, meat, shrimp, lobster, tuna, cheese, eggs, cottage cheese and olives. Add cold-pressed oil, sour cream, natural yogurt or crème fraîche, or make a dressing based on these ingredients. Use erythritol and not sugar if you need to sweeten the dressing.
- **Dinner leftovers**: Leftovers from dinner are an excellent lunch that you can take to work in a container.
- **Bread**: If you want to eat bread for lunch, you should cut slices as thinly as you can. You can garnish the bread with leftovers from the breakfast omelette, but you shouldn't eat cereal grains for both these meals, because then it will be difficult to limit yourself to 50–70 grams of carbohydrates per day. You'll find recipes for good bread replacements with few carbohydrates later in the book.

Dinner

- **Protein and fat sources**: As far as possible, eat unprocessed foods like meat, offal, fish, shellfish, poultry and eggs. Use butter, cold-pressed oils and unsweetened dairy products in food preparation. Try to avoid ready-made fish balls, fish pudding, fish fingers, fish gratin, meatballs, sausages, bread-crumbed foods and ready-to-eat meals. They contain carbohydrates and various additives that are not good for us. If you still want such foods now and then, you should read the ingredients carefully and choose those with the lowest carbohydrate content.

- *Reduce your carbohydrates*: That means cutting down on potatoes, pasta and bread for dinner. Use instead a little basmati rice, wild rice, brown rice or low carb bread. If you want to have potatoes, you shouldn't eat more than 100–150 grams (corresponds to 15–22 grams carbohydrates). Try to eat some meals without traditional starchy foods.
- *Vegetables*: Eat as many vegetables as you wish. You can have lightly boiled, stir-fried or oven-baked vegetables, plus salads to accompany your meat, fish and poultry.
- *Pulses*: Potatoes, rice and pasta can be replaced with lentils, beans and chickpeas in moderate portions.

If you need extra meals

- *Nuts and fruit*: Some unsalted nuts and a small piece of fruit, a carrot or a slice of swede.
- *Fruit and sour cream, crème fraîche, natural yogurt or cottage cheese*: Always eat fruit accompanied by some fat and/or protein – the blood sugar increase will be less.
- *Dinner leftovers*: Easy and good.
- *Eggs*: Scrambled eggs and smoked salmon, omelettes, boiled eggs or a couple of fried eggs – remember vegetables.
- *Cheese*: Some slices of cheese and vegetables.

- **Ham and cheese**: Roll some ham and cheese slices into a couple of lettuce leaves.
- **Vegetables and dip**: Use natural yogurt, sour cream or crème fraîche seasoned with spices – guacamole is easy to make, if healthy and it tastes good.

Alcohol

I'm not much concerned about calories when it comes to low carb food. The exception is alcohol, because alcohol often appears as an addition to the food we eat and doesn't fill us up in the same way as food. In addition, the body prioritises the metabolism of alcohol, so that fat metabolism comes to a halt. Therefore, drink little alcohol if you want to lose weight.

- **Wine** contains 1–3 grams of carbohydrates per 100 ml. A half bottle of red wine contains approximately 350 kcal.
- **Lager** contains 3.2 grams of carbohydrates per 100 ml – i.e. a pint contains approximately 16 grams. The energy per pint is 195 kcal. Pilsner provides a considerable increase in blood sugar and corresponding secretion of insulin which stimulates fat storage. This is the reason that beer drinkers often get a "beer belly". Several types of low carb beer have come onto the market, such as Marstons Low C, Bindings Diat Pils, Miller Light and Michelob Ultra. These have 60–80 % fewer carbohydrates and, consequently, provide a smaller increase in blood sugar and fewer calories.
- **Brandy** contains 2 grams of carbohydrates per 100 ml but the energy amount is 243 kcal per 100 ml. Always use a mixer without sugar.

- **Fortified wine and liqueurs** contain a lot of sugar and should be drunk only on special occasions.

Use of fat in cooking

For frying, it's best to use animal fat such as lard, tallow, duck or goose fat, clarified butter (ghee), butter or cold-pressed vegetable oils with a lot of saturated and mono-unsaturated fatty acids such as coconut oil, olive oil and canola oil. Oils which consist of a lot of saturated and mono-unsaturated fatty acids tolerate high temperatures better than oils that mainly contain polyunsaturated fatty acids. Always check that *cold-pressed* is on the bottle. Coconut oil tolerates heat best because it principally contains saturated fat. Because of the high content of mono-unsaturated fat, olive oil and canola oil tolerate quick frying relatively well. Most of the other cooking oils that are commonly sold are unsuited to frying because they contain mostly poly-unsaturated fatty acids. Frying converts these fatty acids into substances detrimental to health.

Planning your daily routine

With busy daily routines, it is wise to plan the next day's meals the day before. Otherwise, it is too easy just to pop into a shop after work, a little stressed and hungry. Plan your purchases and make sure that you have a selection of the following foods available at home:

- Fresh vegetables, especially those which grow above the ground.
- Eggs – it's practical to have some hard-boiled eggs ready in the refrigerator.
- Meat cold cuts such as ham, smoked pork loin and roast

beef – avoid products containing starch, such as saveloy.
- Bacon – pork that hasn't been smoked is healthier, but start generally with bacon.
- Tinned ham, chicken and turkey.
- Shrimp, lobster tail, fish spread such as hot-smoked mackerel, smoked salmon, tinned sardines, tuna and mackerel.
- Natural cultured milk, cottage cheese, natural yogurt.
- Whipping cream, butter, cold-pressed coconut oil, sour cream, crème fraîche, real mayonnaise.
- Good low carb cheeses.
- Low carb crisp bread.
- Home-made low carb bread or other low carb bread from the shop.
- Have chicken, meat, fish, shellfish, vegetables and berries available in the freezer.
- Olives and cold-pressed olive oil.
- Various types of spices and herbs, fresh and dried.
- Various types of unsalted nuts and seeds.
- Dark chocolate made of least 70 % cacao.

Ketogenic diet

A ketogenic diet is recommended for people with a BMI over 30, high blood pressure, insulin resistance and diabetes. The consumption of carbohydrates should be 20–40 grams per day at most. The advantages of a ketogenic diet are efficient fat metabolism and rapid weight reduction. Hunger and craving for sweets disappear and the energy level increases. The disadvantage is that food choice is limited. Foods such as regular bread, rice, pasta, potatoes and fruit are, for the most part, excluded.

Most people toady eat a mixed diet of carbohydrates, fat and proteins. Consuming high carb foods results in a high production of insulin which stimulates fat storage, inhibits fat metabolism and results in a craving for sweets and high carb foods. With a ketogenic diet, the body is supplied with very few carbohydrates, and the amount of insulin in the blood will therefore decrease. This inhibits efficient fat storage and facilitates fat metabolism. A ketogenic diet inhibits appetite and the desire for sweets.

What happens if the body doesn't get sugar?

During a fast or while switching to a low carb diet, your metabolism gradually switches from using glucose as the most important energy source to using fatty acids and ketone bodies, which are produced from breaking down fatty acids. After a few days of eating very few carbohydrates, you enter ketosis. That means that you are producing so many ketones that some are being excreted in the urine and some via the lungs. Ketone bodies in the urine can be confirmed with ketosis sticks, which can be purchased at a pharmacy. The exhaled air acquires a special smell because of excreted acetone, which is one of the ketone bodies. This kind of ketosis is not dangerous, in contrast to the ketosis that diabetics can develop because of too little insulin and a high blood sugar. Normally it takes three to four weeks before the blood's concentration of ketone bodies reaches a stable level. Ketone bodies and fatty acids create energy using enzymes other than glucose, and therefore some time is needed for the body accustom itself to a low carb diet.

Many people believe that the brain can use only glucose as fuel. It's correct that those who eat a lot of carbohydrate-rich food in the short term are dependent on glucose to cover the brain's requirements, while sleeping, for example. At night, the liver's store of glycogen is reduced in order to meet this need. When the liver's store is nearly depleted, proteins from the muscles are broken down into amino acids, and of these, the liver can convert half to glucose. In addition, the liver breaks down fat into free fatty acids and glycerol, and the glycerol part is converted to glucose. This means that the brain is supplied with glucose throughout the whole night.

The energy supply to the brain changes when the diet contains few carbohydrates, or when we fast for a certain length of time. In both instances, we will have access to free fatty acids and ketones from blood and fatty tissue. Both can be used by the muscles, while ketones can be used by the brain as a replacement for most of the glucose it "normally" uses. Metabolism remains about the same all day long remains whether one is fasting or eating a low carb diet. In starvation, fasting or a ketogenic diet, glucose covers only a quarter of the brain's total energy requirement. In the liver, ketones are produced from fatty acids, enabling the muscles to save protein otherwise used to make glucose. In other words, when you eat more fat and/or metabolise your own fat, you maintain more muscle mass.

Adapting to a ketogenic diet

When you eat a lot of carbohydrates, your metabolism is adapted to glucose. If, on the other hand, you get a large share of energy from fat (your own fat, as well as from food), your metabolism is adapted to fat. It takes time for the body to rearrange itself from one energy source to another. During the transition period, one's energy and ability to perform will be diminished, because the enzyme systems are not adapted to either task. Common symptoms during transition to a ketogenic diet include fatigue, increased urination, increased perspiration, dizziness and headaches. The unpleasantness generally disappears after a few days or weeks, and most people gradually get more energy than they had before. From experience, there is a big difference in how swiftly different people adapt to a new diet. As a rule, it is easier the younger you are.

VLCD – Very Low Calorie Diet

VLCD is a diet which contains 450–800 kcal per day. The VLCD I use contains approximately 700 kcal per day, and the carbohydrate content is approximately 40 grams daily, divided between five VLCD products. It is, as such, a low carb, ketogenic diet. Sometimes these diets are also called "protein-saving fasting diets", because muscle mass is preserved because of sufficient protein intake, while energy is generally taken from the body's own fat stores, as in fasting. When ketosis occurs within the course of a few days, the feeling of hunger diminishes/disappears because the body is getting enough energy from its own fat reserves. The products, which contain all necessary nutrients, consist of a powder you stir into water or milk. The varied menu includes things like different soups, cakes, beverages and energy bars. I often advise mineral and vitamin supplements, but this is an individual evaluation, based on previous diet and blood tests. In addition to the products, plenty of low carb vegetables are included. VLCD results in rapid weight loss and can be a good start for someone who is extremely overweight. Gradually the products are replaced with ordinary low carb containing more fat.

A VLCD must not be used by children and young

people who are growing, pregnant women, lactating women, patients with certain heart disorders, cancer, mental illness, kidney and liver disease or other serious illness. Individual evaluations must be made by the attending physician. A VLCD is used for people with a BMI > 30, but it can also be used with a lower BMI where it is called for. The type of VLCD that I use requires monitoring by a physician.

How long can I be in ketosis?

It's not dangerous to be in ketosis over a long period. Some thrive excellently on a diet of only 20–40 grams of carbohydrates, while others need a little more to feel well. If your weight loss stops for several weeks while you're trying to lose weight, it can helpe to alternate between periods eating a ketogenic diet and periods eating a few more carbohydrates. After completed ketosis, a few more carbohydrates can gradually be introduced. If you consume more than you can tolerate, it's very likely that you'll gain weight again. Each person must therefore find their own tolerance level through trial and error.

Be sure to get regular medical follow-ups

A ketogenic diet is especially useful for people who are overweight and have insulin resistance and/or type 2 diabetes, but it is also useful if you have various nerve disorders like epilepsy. If you have type 2 diabetes and use blood-sugar medication, you must be monitored by your physician, so that you can reduce your dosages as you go. This also applies if you have other chronic disorders, and especially if the disease is being treated with medication. Children, pregnant women and people with type 1 diabetes, kidney failure, liver failure, serious heart rhythm disorders, unstable angina pectoris, eating disorders or mental illnesses must be monitored by a physician in the event of a radical reduction in carbohydrate consumption.

In the event of obesity and ailments or related illness like high blood pressure and low metabolism, I strongly recommend a regular medical consultation, so that the weight reduction can be conducted safely. It's not easy to lose weight – follow-up is therefore very important for maintaining the motivation. Get the information you need to understand what is happening with your body. This makes it easier to maintain your weight after you have achieved your weight loss. Scientific studies show that people who get regular medical follow-up succeed to a much greater degree than those who lose weight on their own.

Exercise

We are designed for motion. Daily movement contributes to a healthier, stronger and more flexible body. Some people love to exercise and gladly do it five times a week, though they are the exception. Others exercise two or three times a week because they feel that they need to in order to preserve their health and a good appearance. A great many don't exercise at all, or do so only periodically.

"The first step is always the hardest" is a good expression that applies to many people – me included. It's difficult to start exercising because there are always good excuses for refraining: housework, shuttling the children, telephoning friends, paying bills, writing e-mails and the like. But exercise is very good for both the body and soul. It makes us feel that we've done something important, and gives us a clear conscience. Many people start to exercise because they feel they must take responsibility for their own health, but the main reason they continue is that it feels good and provides more energy for the daily routine.

Exercise at your own level. Physical activity is especially important if you are overweight or have diabetes, but you shouldn't do hard training if you are extremely heavy. It will be a great burden on your heart and joints and can result in injury. Go on easy walks instead.

We constantly read in newspapers, magazines and books, about training regimes adapted for overweight people, but it isn't so easy for someone who weighs 150 kilograms (23 stone 9) to exercise. People of normal weight can just think what it feels to run around with a backpack weighing 70–80 kilograms (11–13 stone) on their back. If you have insulin resistance, it will be difficult to lose weight just by exercising. You must change your diet at the same time. Which is what Swedish journalist Sten Sture Skaldeman experienced. First he ate his way down some ten's of kilos, and then he *wanted* to exercise.

If you are extremely overweight, I therefore recommend that you reduce your weight with the help of a diet before you start thinking about exercise. Changing diet requires extra planning, so keep your focus on food in the first round. Of course, it's fine if you walk a few times each week at a comfortable tempo. You'll probably be wanting to move more once the first stage of your weight reduction is complete. A person who has lost 20–30 kilograms (3–4 stone) will literally be feeling lighter and will gladly get out the bicycle or the running shoes. The lighter you become, the easier it is to focus on exercising, which also makes it possible to maintain or increase muscle mass. A large muscle mass is favourable, because it requires more energy all day long, also while at rest, and especially if it is used frequently. And exercise is good for self-esteem; most very overweight people have always felt that they can't participate in activities others take for granted.

If you lose a lot of weight, your skin may become too large for your body. Exercise gives good blood circulation, and it stimulates the repair work that the skin needs to adapt itself more easily to your new body.

When exercise has become a part of the daily routine, I recommend strength training with weights. If you haven't done this before, it can be smart to request an hour or two with an instructor at a gym, so that you learn to do the exercises correctly from the start. Strength training with weights is especially important for someone who has insulin resistance and diabetes, because muscle building reduces the insulin resistance. The extent of insulin resistance depends on the relationship of stomach fat to muscle mass: the more stomach fat relative to muscle mass, the more insulin resistance. When muscle mass increases, the need for insulin declines, and when there is less insulin present, it's easier to metabolise fat by exercising. In this way, the fat mass gets smaller at the same time as the muscle mass is being built up.

Regular and hard exercise also reduces insulin resistance independently of its effect on muscle mass. This makes you more insulin sensitive – whether it is injected or comes from the pancreas. The result is that insulin gradually brings down your blood sugar more efficiently. If you're injecting insulin, you'll gradually need smaller doses. The American physician Richard Bernstein, who himself has type 1 diabetes, reports that it takes about two weeks with of hard, daily training to achieve a consistent level of insulin sensitivity. This effect continues for about two weeks after stopping an exercise program. This is particularly important for people who inject insulin. If you stop exercising for several weeks, you'll probably notice that you need higher doses of insulin. Even though you're not training particularly hard, any form of exercise will be beneficial if you're struggling with high blood sugar.

According to normal calorie cocunting, if you weigh 90 kilograms (14 stone 2), you'll lose about 1 kilogram (2 pounds) a week if you daily go for a two-hour walk at a quick pace, with no increase in your food consumption. But as I've mentioned earlier, calorie counting isn't suited for everyone. I have many patients who have exercised harder than this without having lost any weight on a carbohydrate-rich low fat diet. In my opinion, this is due to the high insulin level which inhibits fat metabolism. An equal amount of exercise on a low carb diet on the other hand, is rewarded with significant weight loss.

One advantage with exercise is that many people have less desire to overeat. The reason for this is probably that endorphins, called the body's own morphine, are produced in the brain during exercise. Endorphins can lift the mood and reduce pain and the longing for carbohydrates.

Some people, especially those who eat high carb foods, become extremely hungry when they train. This results in them eating more food and consequently no weight loss despite all their training. Studies show that people who have good exercise habits while losing weight, manage better to remain stable after the weight loss period itself is over.

Exercise influences blood sugar, which most people who take blood sugar medication know. Moderate to hard exercise triggers a stress reaction in the body which results hormonal changes. For example, the levels of cortisol, glucagon, adrenalin and growth hormone increase. These hormones signal the liver and muscles to send sugar to the bloodstream by converting stored glycogen to glucose. A healthy person will react to such hormonal changes by releasing small amounts of stored insulin from the pancreas in order to prevent the blood sugar from rising. The blood sugar will rise, therefore, only slightly and then normalise itself. People with type 2 diabetes react a little differently, because they often lack the rapid secretion of insulin. Their blood sugar will, therefore, increase until the pancreas finally delivers more insulin and gets the blood sugar down again. Thus short-term, strenuous exercise can elevate blood sugar, while long-lasting exercise can lower it.

It's very important that people who use blood sugar-reducing medication, and especially those who use insulin, learn the various effects exercising has on the need for insulin. If not, they risk many periods of low or high blood sugar, and these problems can greatly reduce the pleasure of exercise. If you have various physical problems, I recommend that you talk with your doctor about which type of exercise can be appropriate for you.

Self empowerment

Many studies show that a positive mental attitude has great significance for good health. There have also been many books written about the power of thought and its importance on our ability to accomplish what we want to do. You can look upon your brain as a computer into which you can put lots of information into, and from which you get results that agree whith what you put in. If you constantly think negatively, the brain will enter into a negative mode of thinking, and the consequence will often be negative actions. If, on the other hand, you think positive thoughts, you strengthen the brain's positive hinking, which leads to positive actions.

You will have noticed this many times. Think of a day you overslept. The whole day starts wrong, you think unpleasent thoughts, get irritated in traffic, make sour comments when you arrive at work. You won't get many cheerful comments from anyone that day. Think of another day when you wake up fresh and feeling well, the sun shines, you're happy and pleased with life and you give compliments to colleagues at work. Consequently, you get positive feedback. When you go home, you start up work you have been putting off. I think you know where I'm headed – positive thoughts make us feel better, and we get stronger and better at doing what we want to do. Therefore it's important that you talk nicely to yourself when you are going to change lifestyle. Praise yourself for everything you accomplish. Talk about your project to friends and family. They will, in all probability, give you support and encouragement. Cultivate all positive feedback you get and bring it forth in your memory every time you need it.

When you have a bad day and want to forget the whole project, try to talk with someone who's fond of you and wants to help you accomplish your goal. If you're overweight and want to lose weight, think about how it feels to be slim and look at pictures of yourself when you were slimmer than now. Visualise the goal instead of complaining or being ashamed. It can also be useful to read books on the subject or to communicate with someone on the Internet.

We all know that changing habits is difficult. So, use these tools actively – they will help you. If you want to learn more about such techniques, I advise you to find a good book on the subject or take a course. It really does matter what you say to yourself and to others. Try turning your thoughts about your own body, food, health and your goals in a positive direction.

Realistic expectations

Unrealistic expectations are an important reason why many overweight people abandon their attempt to lose weight. Perhaps you read stories with happy endings in the magazines about people who achieve quick results. If you yourself lose only 2 kilograms (4 pounds) in a month, you may get disappointed and think it's not worth the effort. If you ever catch yourself thinking like this, remember the following:

- Extremely overweight people often lose weight faster than slightly overweight people. One of the reasons for this is that they have bodies which require more energy, and body that has plenety of fat gives up weight more easily.
- Men lose weight faster than women, partly because they're larger as a rule and have more muscle mass.
- Younger people often lose weight faster than older people, again because they often have more muscle mass, a faster metabolism, and they have a more active lifestyle.
- People who have never dieted before often lose weight faster than so-called yo-yo dieter.
- People who have a lot of fluid in the body lose weight rapidly because they're excreting water.
- Weight can increase in the short-term because of fluid retention – which is often the case with hormonal swings during the course of woman's menstrual cycle, after training, and after consuming a lot of salt and sugar/starch.
- People who use medication lose weight more slowly, because some medication affects the appetite and/or the metabolism.

- Furthermore, people are different. We just have to accept that – however unfair it may seem.

Even though you might not be losing weight rapidly, it doesn't mean that you're doing anything wrong. Be patient – it doesn't matter whether you take six months or two years to reach your goal. Look at this as a long-term lifestyle change to achieve good health, not as a short-term diet to lose weight. The most important thing is that you reach your goal, and that you have a life worth living. If you continue steadily with your new diet, you'll get the results you want. Perhaps you've dieted many times, and the only result was that you weighed more than before? It's not good to lose weight too rapidly, because the body has to make many adjustments along the way. Your skin, for example, looks much better if you lose weight more slowly. It has time to tighten up and adjust to your new body. With faster weight loss, the skin isn't able to this. Later, if surplus skin causes problems, plastic surgery may have to be considered.

Sooner or later, many people will arrive at a so-called plateau. This means that weight loss stops for a while. If the body has lost ten kilograms (a stone or two), it "needs" to evaluate the situation. "Dare I let go of more fat now, or will I need the fat in case of a food shortage?" Several weeks can go by before the body again decides to let go of more weight. When you reach a plateau, you must carry on as before. If your weight doesn't budge over a long period, try increasing your carbohydrate consumption for a couple of weeks and then restrict it again – this often helps. You should also consider your portion sizes – gradually, as the body becomes smaller, it will need less food.

There are some serious obstacles to losing weight, and they are as follows:

- **High consumption of alcohol:** Alcohol contains energy which often comes in addition to the food we eat. When you drink alcohol, the liver sets to metabolising alcohol instead of fat. Alcohol is toxic to the body, and the liver wants to get rid of it as rapidly as possible. This means that alcohol can block the break down of your fat stores. Furthermore, many people lose control when they drink alcohol, and they decide to eat more chocolate, cakes or potato crisps. High alcohol consumption over a long period can lead to a fatty liver and later to liver damage. This, in turn, results in alcohol being broken down more slowly than before.

- *Stress:* Many people put on weight when they're exposed to stress. This is due to the hormone cortisol, which leads to elevated blood sugar and subsequently to elevated insulin, so that you store fat more efficiently. This can occur even though you're eating the same as – or even less than – before. Other people lose control over what they put in their mouths when they are exposed to stress. They don't have time to plan the day, and then their diet can quickly turn to fast food and pizza. The result of inadequate planning can be a rapid weight increase, which only leads to yet more stress.

- *Cortisone:* This medication works well on various inflammatory conditions and pain. However, it results in the same problems as too much self-produced cortisol and is a real hindrance to weight loss. If you have to use cortisone, you should try, in cooperation with your doctor, to find your way to the smallest effective dose.

Eat enough food

If you want to lose weight, it's more important that you eat the right food than that you eat little food. If you eat small quantities, you may lose weight for a time, but you'll quickly gain it back when you return to former diet. If you eat too little food over a long period, the body may react in the same way as it did thousands of years ago. It thinks there's a food shortage, and that you'll starve. The body will then start saving its fat reserves to ensure enough energy to survive. Instead of burning only the fat, the body also consumes muscle tissue. It is of course very costly for the body to have a large muscle mass, because muscles require a lot of energy. In other words: if you reduce a lot of weight by eating little food, you'll lose muscle mass. Then when you can't handle starving yourself any longer, you'll put on fat, and the result becomes less muscle mass, poor metabolism and greater fat mass.

What should I eat when I'm at a party?

If you have weight problems, I think you should talk to your family, friends and colleagues about your new diet – most of them will understand that you need to do something for your health. Take along some food you *can* eat, which you can even share with the other guests.

Sometimes, you have to be a little tactical when you are eating with other people. Let's say you're at a party where there are appetisers with bread, potatoes, a sweet dessert and then cake with coffee. Nobody will notice if you avoid the bread and potatoes; it's often easiest to avoid these foods. You can take a small potato for the sake of appearances and eat half of it. If you think it's hard not having dessert, you can take a little and eat half of that. When coffee is served, have a cup of coffee without cake. If you feel that you're being impolite, take a thin piece and leave some on the dessert plate. You'll reduce your carbohydrate consumption considerably this way. It's also important that you don't indulge the craving for sweets you may get once you get home. You will, in any case, be going back to your chosen regime the next day.

What should I eat when I'm travelling?

When you're travelling, always plan what you're going to eat – whether that means dining out or taking a packed lunch along with you. If you haven't planned your day and you get hungry, you'll have to resort to temporary solutions – and that can be tricky! Buy a hot dog or hamburger but ask them to hold the bread. Or why not try a kebab, where you eat the contents and leave the bread behind? In shops that have fresh produce, you can buy salads with meat and cheese, ready-cooked chicken, beef patties and omelettes. At hotels, as a rule, there's plenty of low carb food you can enjoy. There's often a buffet, which makes it easy to choose right. At restaurants, tell the waiter what you want to have – after all, it's you who is paying! It can be a good idea to choose a specific dish and ask to have the potatoes exchanged with vegetables.

Low carb diet
if you don't have weight problems

Perhaps you're thinking: is a low carb diet beneficial for a person who is slim and has never had problems with weight? Indeed it is! A low carb diet is good for most of us. As you have seen from the case histories, not everyone had a weight problem, but nevertheless they had problems related to what they were eating.

Acid reflux

A great many people suffer from acid reflux, but they generally get rid of it when they quit eating regular bread and other carbohydrates. Acid reflux is usually due to eating things your stomach doesn't tolerate. If you have smoked for many years, you probably know that your lungs have not been pleased with all the toxins they are getting every day. Well, the stomach works exactly the same way. Pharmacists sell a huge amount of drugs for acid reflux. If you don't want to be part of that statistic, I recommend switching to a low carb diet. I hear regularly from my patients that they have quit using such drugs when they change their diet.

Gas and stomach pain

Many people are bothered by a bloated stomach, even if they aren't overweight. Their gas problem is due to the fact that sugar ferments in the intestines, creating a lot of gas that has to be expelled. Besides pain and discomfort, you may be having to release gas constantly, which isn't always convenient. And of course there is often an unpleasant odour. You will, allmost certainly, avoid this problem by reducing your consumption of carbohydrates. Many of my patients report that although they passed gas constantly before, they can't remember the last time it happened.

Constipation and diarrhoea

This is a very common problem. Many people have loose bowel several times a day, while others are constipated and defecate only a couple of times each week. They also often get haemorrhoids. Which results in itching and pain around the anus. Why some people get diarrhoea and others constipation on a typical modern diet isn't easy to say. Patients who describe these problems often eat about the same type of food. But, as we have seen, people are different, and some react with diarrhoea and others with constipation when the intestine is being treated poorly.

It is nevertheless my experience that these patients function normally on low carb food. During a transition period, some may become constipated, but it usually passes. If you get constipated at the start of a low carb diet, it is probably because the intestine has been accustomed to getting a lot of fibre that irritates the intestine, making it want to eject the stool as quickly as possible. If constipation is a problem, you should eat a lot of fat, fibrous vegetables, flax seeds or psyllium and drink plenty of water. Daily physical activity is also important.

Today's diet doesn't contribute to an intestinal flora with good intestinal bacteria. It may therefore be beneficial to take lactic acid bacteria in the form of tablets or capsules. Eating a low carb diet with a lot of natural food, it's very likely that you will eventually achieve good intestinal health, and your stool will become almost odour free.

Skin, hair and nails

Blemished skin with pimples and blackheads is a common problem among adults as well as children. Dry hair with split ends, hair loss and cracked nails are also very common. People customarily remedy these problems with a myriad of creams, shampoos, conditioners and nail polish, but such measures don't remove the cause of the problem. Instead of treating what you see, you should eat right, so that your body has enough nutrients to give you healthy skin, strong nails and nice hair. Which is not what the body prioritises if you lack nutrients, or if you ingest things you shouldn't have. Having nice skin is, of course, not vital. But having internal organs that function right is, so they get priority. One of the skin's jobs is to excrete unwanted substances. The fewer unnatural foods you eat, the less waste has to go out through the skin. A varied low carb diet gives you more natural fat and more vitamins and minerals than a typical modern diet, and gradually the body will get enough nutrients to take care of the skin, hair and nails.

Pain in the muscles and bones

Many people have pain in their muscles and bones without being overweight or having had injuries or serious illnesses. This is often due to inflammations because of too much insulin, too many omega-6 fatty acids and too little omega-3. My experience is that these pains disappear on a low carb diet with natural food. Patients who go to a physiotherapist or have massages often report that the therapist comments on how flexible they have become in their musculature after changing their diet.

Eczema and psoriasis

These are common disorders which many people have without being particularly sick or heavy. The cause is often the same as mentioned before. Many patients tell me that the eczema they have had for years disappeared in the course of a few weeks after they changed their diet. The same applies for psoriasis.

Gingivitis

There are certainly many who have infected gums without being overweight, and there is probably not much doubt that it is from eating too much non-nutritious, sweet food. People who eat natural food seldom get gingivitis, and you don't need to either.

Get-up-and-go

We live in a hectic society and we have a lot we want to do with our lives. Nearly everyone wishes that they had more energy. I can almost guarantee you that you will on a low carb diet. Some people have less drive the first week after the change, but then they notice that things are going better and better. It's important to eat enough natural fat to have a lot of energy.

Sleep

Sleep problems are common. The obvious reasons are that you're up until long into the night and sleep during the day, so that you can't get to sleep again at night, or that you drink a lot of coffee or alcohol in the evening. A glass of wine doesn't hurt, but large quantities of alcohol often result in poor sleep quality and waking too early. Many people wake at night because blood sugar is low, and they experience that if they have a glass of milk, a banana or the like they fall asleep again. You won't wake at night because of low blood sugar when you have a stable blood sugar eating a low carb diet. On this diet, your sleep will also be of better quality and you'll need less.

Mood

Fluctuating moods and moody people are not uncommon.

Some people will always be moody for one reason or another, but with a stable blood sugar level most people's mood actually becomes more stable. Many become irritated during the period before eating, and they get very cranky. This is often due to low blood sugar, which has a negative effect the brain. So my recommendation is making sure to eat food that doesn't keep your blood sugar and your mood on a rollercoaster ride.

Children

Most people have probably seen children at a birthday party after eating a lot of cakes and sweets. They go right through the roof – right? It's because their blood sugar is so high – it does something to their brain. This is no doubt a sensible mechanism in so far as blood sugar goes down as a result of high physical activity. You've probably heard that children with ADHD become far calmer when they eat fewer sugary foods.

Children need to grow and develop, and for that they need plenty of fat and proteins that also contain essential nutrients that the body can't make itself. These nutrients are found in foods such as meat, fish, shellfish, poultry, buts, seeds, cold-pressed oils, eggs and unsweetened milk products. If children have plenty of these foods, they stay full for longer and have less need to constantly be eating slices bread and sugary foods.

Heavy menstrual bleeding

A great many women bleed heavily when they menstruate. After changing their diet, my female patients report shorter and less painful menstruation, with less bleeding.

Recipes

It is one thing to have recipe books on the shelf, but it's another thing to put them to good use in everyday bustle. In daily life, most people prepare food on a regular routine. Here I provide some recipes that can easily be varied, so that you will always have some ideas on hand. Many people miss bread when they are to start on a low carb diet. This is not something we *must* eat, but here I offer some good alternatives. When "oil" appears in the recipes, it must always be cold-pressed. You can purchase ingredients marked with * in health food shops.

For more tips, visit www.thescandinaviandiet.com

Bread and bread substitutes

HIGH PROTEIN BREAD
Makes 1 loaf

You can use whole or crushed flax seeds. Whole flax seeds are good for the functioning of the intestine, while crushing the seeds makes the nutrients in them available for absorption.

4 eggs
½ container crème fraîche or quark (dry curd cottage cheese)
3 tbs oil
1 tbs baking powder
50 g (1.75 oz) flax seeds
60 g (2 oz) wheat bran
50 g (1.75 oz) sesame seeds
50 g (1.75 oz) sunflower seeds

Whip the eggs slightly and blend in the crème fraîche or quark and cold-pressed oil. Add the dry ingredients and mix well. The dough should have a soft consistency, like a thick porridge. If it seems a little thin, add a few more seeds or wheat bran.

Line a 30 x 12 cm (5 x 11 inches), bread pan with baking paper. Put the dough in the pan and bake the bread on the lowest rack at 180 °C (350 °F) for 55 minutes. Let it cool before serving.

This bread should be kept in the refrigerator. It can be frozen.

Variation: You can add a pinch of salt, a pinch of crushed caraway, or some herbs. The seeds can be ground to flour rather than being used whole. Some of the bran can be replaced with ground almonds that you can purchase in health food shops or make yourself by grinding almonds finely. Some of the seeds can be replaced with chopped walnuts. You can use less baking powder – try different ways. 1 portion makes a low loaf, while a double portion makes a normal size loaf. If you are making a large loaf, bake it for 10 minutes longer.

OPTIMAL BREAD

Makes 1 loaf

10 large eggs
100 g (3.5oz) coarse or fine spelt flour
1 tbs baking powder
1 pinch salt
1 pinch pepper
50 g (1.75 oz) oat bran
100 g (3.5 oz) sunflower seeds
100 g (3.75 oz) melted butter

Separate the eggs. Whip the egg whites stiff and add the egg yolks one at a time while you continue to whip. Add the flour together with the baking powder, salt and pepper. Then, add oat bran and sunflower seeds and finally the melted butter.

Mix well and put the dough into a baking paper-lined bread pan of approximately 30 x 12 cm (5 x 11 inches). Bake the bread on the lowest rack in the oven at 220 °C (425 °F), until it has turned a golden-brown colour.

Let the bread cool on a rack and store it in the refrigerator packed in cling-film or paper. It can be frozen.

Variation: If you don't have spelt flour, you can use regular wheat flour.

LOW CARB BARS

The mixture will fill a large roasting tray

5 eggs
250 g (9 oz) sunflower seeds

250 g (9 oz) sesame seeds
250 g (9 oz) crushed flax seeds
250 g (9 oz) chopped walnuts
1 tsp salt

Mix all the ingredients and spread the mixture onto a greased roasting tray. Bake it in the middle of the oven at 190 °C (375 °F) for 10–11 minutes.

Leave to cool and then cut into bars of your desired size. They can be stored in the refrigerator for 4–5 days. They are well-suited to freezing and will thaw in only a few minutes.

Variation: The quantity of the various seeds can be varied according to what you have and like. The total quantity must, however, be as specified above.

BREAKFAST MIX

200 g (7 oz) sunflower seeds
200 g (7 oz) flax seeds
200 g (7 oz) pumpkin seeds
200 g (7 oz) sesame seeds chopped, unsalted almonds, nuts or coconut if you like!

Mix all the ingredients.

Store the breakfast mix in a tight container. Serve it with berries and natural cultured milk, cottage cheese, natural yogurt or coconut milk.

Variation: If you don't have berries and want a sweet taste, sprinkle a little erythritol on top. If you want some grain in your mixture, it's best to use rolled oats or rye, barley or spelt flakes.

PANCAKE

Makes 1 portion

2 eggs
2 tbs cottage cheese
2 tbs rolled oats
1 tbs cinnamon

Mix all the ingredients into a batter and fry the pancake in a frying pan on low heat as you would an omelette.

You can have berries, grated apple or erythritol on the pancake.

Variation: Instead of cinnamon, you can use cacao or cardamom. Rolled oats can be exchanged with flax, sesame or sunflower seeds. The pancake can be used for breakfast, lunch or supper. Some people make waffles from this batter – you just have to try this on your own.

CHEESE PANCAKES

Makes about 8 pieces

3 eggs
¼ container drained quark
150–200 g (5.25 – 7 oz) grated cheese
Salt and white pepper.
Herbs as desired, such as basil, thyme, oregano, garlic.

Separate the egg whites and yolks. Beat the eggs whites stiff – they will get stiffer if you add a pinch of salt – and put them aside.

Mix the egg yolks and quark with a spoon or hand blender. Stir in the grated cheese. Season to taste with salt, white pepper and herbs. Carefully fold in the beaten egg white.

Put small dabs on a baking sheet lined with baking paper – remember that the dough will spread while baking.

Bake the biscuits in the middle of the oven at 175 °C (350 °F) for about 20 minutes, or until they have turned a golden brown colour. Let them cool on a rack.

They can be eaten as they are, or you can put a spread or pizza topping on them. Store them in the refrigerator.

SPINACH MUFFINS

Makes 16 pieces

250 g (9 oz) fresh spinach
140 g (5 oz) feta cheese
1 chopped garlic clove
4 eggs
200 ml (7 fl oz) whipping cream
¼ tsp ground nutmeg
½ tsp fresh-ground pepper
Grated white or yellow cheese

Cook the spinach quickly in a little water until the leaves wilt. Pour off the water.

Mix all the ingredients except for the grated white cheese.

Divide the batter into a greased muffin pan. Alternatively, put the batter in an oven-proof dish and divide it when it has baked. Sprinkle plenty of grated cheese over the muffins and bake them at 175 °C (350 °F) for about 30 minutes, or until the egg mixture has stiffened.

Store the muffins in the refrigerator. They're super to take along for lunch.

Dinner

Stir-frying

There are infinite possibilities with fresh vegetables, various types of meat, poultry, fish and shellfish. Season according to taste. Soy sauce can be the answer if you don't know what to season with!

STIR-FRIED CHICKEN

Makes 1 portion

150–200 g (5.25–7 oz) chicken fillet sliced into 1 cm thick slices
500 g (1 lb 1 oz) broccoli florets
30 g (1 oz) sugar peas
1 coarsely chopped onion
1 tsp grated fresh ginger
4 tbs water
1–2 tsp soy sauce
Oil for frying

Heat plenty of oil in a wok or a pan with non-stick coating. Add the chicken pieces. Turn them often and fry until they have become golden. Add broccoli, sugar peas, onion, ginger and water. Let the whole thing simmer for about 10 minutes. If it gets too dry, you can add a little extra oil. Stir in the soya sauce at the end.

Soups

Soups are good and simple food. A lot of the nutrients from the foods remain in the pot instead of being tossed out with the cooking water. Along with soups you can have low carb bread or cheese pancakes as an accompaniment if you don't get full enough from the soup.

Meat soup

The best thing for making soup is a good stock you have cooked from bones. Actually the bones should be baked for a while first and *then* cooked in water. This is what brings out the real meat flavour. It's not as difficult as it sounds. The most important thing is that you put leftover bones in the freezer instead of throwing them away. One day when you're home, you put the leftover bones in a large pot and fill with water so that it covers the bones. You can also put in some chopped vegetables such as carrots, celery root, leeks and onions. For herbs, use fresh parsley, thyme and bay leaf – dried herbs also work well. You can also put whole peppercorns and a little salt into the pot. The most important thing of though is that you cook the stock from bones.

When the whole thing has come to a boil, skim off foam and let the stock simmer on low heat for a few hours under a lid. For beef, wild game and sheep bones, let the stock simmer for 5 hours; for pork bones, 3 hours and, poultry bones 1–2 hours.

After cooling, pour the stock into suitable containers. You can use the stock for soup or sauce the same day or the day after, and if you have anything left, simply freeze it again.

If you have a good stock, it's easy to make a good soup. Sauté different vegetables in olive oil or butter in a pot, then pour in the stock and let it come to a boil. If the stock is very fatty, use one-fourth stock and the rest water.

If you don't have a meat stock on hand, use meat bouillon. Put pieces of meat in the soup – if possible from the same animal that you used for the stock. While the soup cooks slowly, season it with what you want. Salt and pepper are basic seasonings. After that, you can decide whether you want to add herbs, or perhaps even some curry powder. If you want to have a richer soup, add whipping cream or crème fraîche.

Fish soup

Make fish soup in the same way as meat soup. Gather together fish bones, fish heads and shrimp shells, which will make an excellent and nutritious stock. Take care that you don't include blood, guts or gills, as this will give the stock a bad taste. Cook the stock for up to 1 hour, no longer, otherwise it may get a sort of cod liver oil, gluey taste.

If you don't have home-made fish stock, use fish bouillon. Sauté different vegetables in olive oil or butter in a pot, add stock and bring it to a boil. Let the stock cook on a low heat until the vegetables are tender. Then add the fish. Bring the soup to a boil, turn down the heat and let the fish simmer until it is cooked. Stir in cream or crème fraîche if you wish. Season to taste with salt, pepper and any other spices you like.

Mushroom soup

Fry as many mushrooms as you want and season them with salt and pepper. Then, add meat bouillon and whipping cream. The more whipping cream you have, the thicker the soup will be. Crème fraîche can also be used.

Soup from mashed vegetables

You can make soup from all kinds of mashed vegetables – for example cauliflower. Cook cauliflower florets until they are tender and then mash them, along with the cooking water, with a hand blender. If you want more taste, add an onion or two that you have sautéed in butter or olive oil. Add whipping cream and spices. If you think you need more taste, crumble a boullion cube into the mixture.

TOMATO SOUP

Makes 4–6 portions

500 g (1 lb 1oz) tomatoes
1 onion
A small amount of fresh, chopped chilli pepper or a pinch of chilli powder
4 tbs olive oil
2 cans chopped tomatoes
1 litre (2 pints) vegetable bouillon
Salt, pepper and herbs, for example basil
Whipping cream – optional
Boiled eggs in quarters, sliced avocadoes, fried or boiled chicken pieces, shrimp

Cut the tomatoes into pieces and chop the onion coarsely. Sauté onion and chilli pepper in olive oil in a frying pan and add the tomato pieces. Then add the tinned tomatoes and the vegetable bouillon. Let the whole thing cook for 15–20 minutes.

Take the pot off the heat and stir the mixture with a hand blender. Season to taste with salt, pepper and herbs. Whipping cream makes the soup richer and milder. To get a little more substance to this soup, serve it with hard-boiled eggs, avocado, pieces of chicken, shrimp or crayfish.

Casseroles

Casseroles consist mainly of vegetables, meat and gravy are easy to make. Use mostly vegetables that grow above ground. Sweet corn contains a lot of carbohydrates, so don't use much of it. Use meat or minced meat instead of sausages and sausage meat. You must *not* thicken the casserole with flour or cornflour. If you use whipping cream and crème fraîche, let it cook only until it has achieved the proper consistency. Alternatively, use a little flax seed meal or vegetable gum which you can buy in health food shops.

LAMB CASSEROLE

Makes 4–6 portions

2 onions sliced thinly
2 garlic cloves, finely chopped
Olive oil for frying
750 g (1 lb 10 oz) trimmed lamb from shoulder or thigh, cubed
salt and pepper
2 tsp herbs de Provence
1 can chopped tomatoes
200 ml (7 fl oz) bouillon
A tiny amount of cornflour if needed

Brown the onion and garlic in oil in a frying pan and transfer it to a pot. Brown the meat cubes with a little salt and pepper and add them to the pot. Then add the herbs de Provence, chopped tomatoes and bouillon.

Let the whole thing simmer under cover on low heat, until the meat is tender, about 30 minutes. Thicken the sauce with a little cornflour mixed in a little water if you think it is too thin. Season to taste with spices.

CHICKEN SALAD

Makes about 4 portions

500 g (1 lb 1 oz) chicken fillet in pieces, fried in olive oil or butter
Mixed greens
1 avocado sliced in cubes and/or plenty of feta cheese
4 tbs pine nuts, sunflower seeds or walnuts
8 cherry tomatoes or regular tomatoes sliced in quarters
1 finely chopped spring onion

Mix all the ingredients. Sprinkle a few pine nuts, walnuts or sunflower seeds on top for garnish.

OIL DRESSING

200 ml (7 fl oz) oil
The juice from half a lemon
Chopped herbs such as oregano, basil, parsley or chive
Salt and pepper
Mustard (optional)

Mix the oil and lemon juice and add the chopped herbs. Season the dressing to taste with salt, pepper and some mustard. Pour the dressing over the salad or is served on the side.

Dinner in an oven-proof dish

An easy way to make dinner is to bake it in the oven. Grease an oven-proof dish with butter or olive oil and fill it with your desired vegetables and meat, poultry or fish. Add a sauce as you like. For a simple sauce use whipping cream and spices. Sprinkle plenty of grated cheese on the top.

SALMON IN AN OVEN-PROOF DISH

Makes 1 portion

Butter or olive oil
150–200 g (5.25 – 7 oz) salmon
5–7 small broccoli florets
½ carrot in slices
¼ leek in rings
4 large mushrooms in slices
Salt, pepper and herbs
Lemon juice and olive oil

Grease the dish and add the salmon and vegetables. Sprinkle on salt, pepper and herbs. Drizzle some lemon juice and plenty of olive oil over the top. Put the dish in the middle of the oven at 175 °C (350 °F) for about 25 minutes.

PIZZA

Size: 1 baking dish

For this pizza, you can use whatever topping you desire, but avoid high carb ingredients such as sweet tomato sauces and sweetcorn.

Base:
8 eggs
1 package of natural Philadelphia cream cheese
½–1 tsp baking powder
About 200 g (7 oz) grated cheese

Oregano and/or garlic powder
About 100 g (3.5 oz) grated cheese to sprinkle on the crust

Mix all the ingredients in a food processor except for 1 dl (3.5 fl oz) of the grated cheese. Pour the batter onto a baking dish lined with baking paper and spread it out. Sprinkle the remaining cheese over it. Bake it low in the oven for about 15 minutes at 200–225 °C (400–450 °F), until it has become slightly golden.

Take the baking dish out of the oven and add the topping you prefer. Bake the pizza until the cheese has melted.

Put it on a rack after baking, or it will become soft.

This pizza tastes great the day after as well. It can be eaten cold or warmed up.

PIZZA OMELETTE

Makes 4 small pizza omelettes

400 g (14 oz) minced meat
1 package of bacon, chopped
A bit of leek in slices
Chopped mushrooms
1 sweet pepper chopped
Olive oil or butter for frying
8 eggs
8 tbs whipping cream
Lots of grated cheese
Pizza spices

Fry the minced meat, bacon, leek, mushrooms and sweet pepper in butter or olive oil in a frying pan.

Blend the eggs and whipping cream together.

Put ¼ of the meat mixture in a small frying pan and pour on ¼ of the egg mixture.

Sprinkle on grated cheese and pizza spices.

Turn the omelette over and fry it a little on the other side as well.

Do the same with the rest of the meat and egg mixture.

PIE WITHOUT PIE DOUGH

Makes 1 pie

200 g (7 oz) diced ham
½ finely chopped onion
1 small leek in thin slices
4 eggs
400 ml (14 fl oz) milk
4 tbs cottage cheese
50 g (1.75 oz) grated cheese

Mix all the ingredients except the grated cheese in a bowl. Grease a pie plate with olive oil and pour in the mixture.

Sprinkle grated cheese on the top and bake the pie in the middle of the oven at 175 °C (350 °F) until the egg mixture has stiffened.

NORWEGIAN SOUR CREAM PORRIDGE ("RØMMEGRØT")

Makes about 2 portions

300 ml (10.5 fl oz) sour cream (try to find the fattest one. If you cannot find higher than 20 % fat, try using double/ clotted cream instead of whipping cream)
100–150 ml (7–10.5 fl oz) whipping cream

100–200 ml (7–14 fl oz) water
1 tsp flax seed meal or vegetable gum (low carb seeds thickening agent)
1 tsp salt
Erythritol*, cinnamon, butter and perhaps cured meats alongside

Bring the sour cream to a boil and let it cook slowly on medium heat for 2–3 minutes.

Mix the whipping cream and a little of the water in a small container with a cover. Add the low carb thickening agent and shake it till it thickens.

Pour the thickening slowly into the boiling sour cream while you stir it together well. If you stir too vigorously, the fat in the cream will separate out.

Let the porridge stand and cook a little more on low to medium heat for 5–10 minutes and stir constantly. If the porridge becomes too thick, you can thin it with a little water or whipping cream to taste. If the sour cream porridge doesn't become thick enough, make a little more thickener and stir it in. But don't use too much because the porridge can quickly become too thick.

Use a hand blender if you get lumps in the porridge.

Season to taste with salt.

Serve the sour cream porridge with erythritol, cinnamon, butter and slices of cured meat if you like.

Side dishes

You can use many of the recipes you already have, but you may have to change your side dishes to your dinner meals. Below I have suggested some alternatives. Eat a salad in addition if possible.

Cooked vegetables

Cook plenty of vegetables such as cabbage, red cabbage, broccoli and cauliflower. You can certainly use frozen vegetables, but preferably not medleys, which usually contain starchy root vegetables and sweetcorn. Vegetables taste especially good with melted butter.

Creamed spinach

Buy frozen spinach in the shop. It's always good to have it in the freezer. You heat up the spinach in a little water and butter. Then, add crème fraîche, whipping cream, or sour cream. Add a generous amount for extra good flavour.

Mashed cauliflower and other mashed vegetables

Chop the cauliflower into small pieces and cook them in a little lightly-salted water until they're tender. Pour off the water. Then mash the cauliflower with a hand blender. Add butter, whipping cream and plenty of grated cheese. If you don't have whipping cream, just use cheese and butter. Season to taste with salt and pepper. If you have some favourite spices, try adding them.

Variation: You can make many types of mashed vegetables, for example, broccoli, carrots, celery root and swedes. Often it's good to blend various vegetables. You can, for example, mix broccoli and cauliflower, swedes and celery root, carrots and cauliflower. Just use your imagination!

Hot vegetable medley

For this dish, use whatever vegetables you have in the house: onions, garlic, leeks, sweet peppers, squash (courgette), carrots and tomatoes. Coarsely chop the vegetables and put butter or olive oil in a large pot or frying pan. It's always smart to sauté the onions until they are transparent first, for they need the longest time. After that, add the other vegetables. Use medium heat and let the vegetables simmer until they have become tender. Stir occasionally. Then, add a can of chopped tomatoes and season with salt, pepper, and whatever herbs you like. If you have time, simmer the mixture on low heat a while; it will taste even better!

Oven-baked vegetables

Use cauliflower or broccoli florets, carrots, sweet peppers, squash (courgette), aubergines, string beans, onions and garlic. Sauté a finely chopped onion and garlic in butter or olive oil in a frying pan. Put the onion mixture into an oven-proof dish and add the other diced vegetables. Sprinkle on salt and pepper. Mix in a tin of chopped tomatoes and put tin foil over the dish. Bake the vegetables in the middle of the oven at 175 °C (350 °F) for about 45 minutes. When there are a few minutes left, sprinkle on some extra nice grated cheese. Remove the foil, put the dish back in the oven and leave it for a few minutes until the cheese has melted. If you think this will take too long, you can cook the vegetables a few minutes first and then bake them in the oven under high heat.

Sautéed courgette

Slice or chop the courgette and sprinkle on salt and pepper. Heat butter or olive oil in a frying pan and sauté the courgette. Squeeze on a little lemon before serving.

Mushrooms

Mushrooms are easy to get hold of all year round and simple to fry with butter, salt and pepper. If you want creamed mushrooms, add whipping cream or crème fraîche and let it cook down a little. Creamed mushrooms taste delicious with meat.

GUACAMOLE

2 ripe avocadoes
1 small onion
2 garlic cloves
½ fresh chilli pepper
The juice of 1 lime
A pinch of salt and pepper

Cut avocado and onion in pieces.

Mix all the ingredients in a blender or with the aid of a hand blender. If you use a mortar or spoon, the onion, garlic and chilli pepper must first be chopped finely. Season the guacamole to taste with salt and pepper.

Smoothies, berries, cakes, desserts, confectionary and snacks

The consumption of sugar should be reduced radically because it damages health. A natural type of sugar called erythritol has now appeared on the market. This sugar substitute doesn't produce an increase in blood sugar or insulin and adds very little energy (0.2 kcal/g). For that reason, I've used erythritol in the recipes that follow.

SMOOTHIES

Breakfast for 1 person

100 g (3.5 oz) fresh or frozen berries
2 eggs

1 handful of nuts or seeds
1–2 tbs room temperature coconut fat
250 ml (10.5 fl oz) natural yogurt, coconut milk, natural cultured milk or water

Mix all the ingredients in a blender. You can also use a hand blender, but then you should chop the nuts in advance. If a sweeter version is needed, you can add erythritol.

Variation: The sky's the limit when you're going to make a smoothie. If you want to make a low carb smoothie, though, remember not to use too many fruit/berries and, instead, use plenty of proteins and fat. Good sources for this are milk products without added sugar, nuts, seeds, eggs, coconut oil, avocadoes, and coconut milk.

BERRY COMPOTE

2 kg (4 lb 7 oz) berries
½ kg (1 lb 1 oz) erythritol (taste your way forth)
1 bag pectin powder (for freezing)

Put the berries in a large bowl and mix in the erythritol combined with pectin powder for freezing. Cut berries, such as strawberries, into smaller pieces or mash them with a hand blender. Then divide the berry compote in freezer bags and freeze what you won't use during the next 3–4 days.

The compote can be stored for only a few days after thawing because there is no preservative added. Use it on low carb bread, pancakes and waffles. It is also good in smoothies and home-made low carb ice cream.

WAFFLES

300 ml (10.5 fl oz) crème fraîche or sour cream
4 eggs
2 tsp baking powder
5–6 tsp low carb thickener such as carob
1 tsp cardamom
1 tbs erythritol
100 g (3.5 oz) melted butter

Whisk all the ingredients into a batter and fry the waffles in butter. They can be eaten as they are, or with berry compote.

ALMOND CAKE WITH BERRIES

Cake:
100 g (3.5 oz) almonds
65 g 2.5 oz) butter
125 ml (4.25 fl oz) whole milk
1 egg
1 ½ t baking powder
85 g (3 oz) erythritol

Filling:
Berries and erythritol

Grind the almonds and put them aside.

Melt the butter and mix in milk. Whisk in the egg with a steel whisk.

Mix the ground almonds, baking powder and erythritol in a large mixing bowl. Add the liquid and mix the batter together well.

Pour the batter into a round pan with a diameter of 20–

26 cm (8–10 inches) or in a pie pan. Distribute the berries on the batter and sprinkle on erythritol.

Bake the cake on a rack in the middle of the oven at 200 °C (400 °F) for about 30 minutes.

Variation: You can push apple pieces down in the dough or use rhubarb instead of berries. The cake can be served with whipped cream. Sliced almonds and grated 70 % chocolate make a great garnish.

PINEAPPLE DESSERT

1 container cottage cheese
2 tbs room temperature coconut fat
½ fresh pineapple cut into pieces
2 tbs shredded coconut

Mix the cottage cheese and coconut fat well. Stir in the pineapple pieces and sprinkle on the coconut.
Variation: You can also try a little finely chopped dark chocolate and chopped nuts on top of the dessert. Other fruits or berries can also be used.

BERRIES AND CREAM

Whipping cream
Erythritol
Berries, thawed or fresh

Whip the cream, while slowly adding in erythritol to taste. Serve the berries with the cream and some chopped nuts or sliced almonds if you like.

STRAWBERRIES WITH CHOCOLATE

70 % chocolate
Fresh strawberries

Melt the chocolate in a double-boiler. Dip the strawberries in the chocolate and let them cool.

CHOCOLATE ICE CREAM

Makes 6–8 portions

5 eggs
8 tbs erythritol
500 ml (about a pint) whipping cream
100 g (3.5 oz) 70 % chocolate

Beat the eggs and erythritol together till yellow and fluffy. Whip the whipping cream until it is quite stiff. Melt the chocolate in a double-boiler. Fold the egg mixture and the cream together carefully and then stir in the melted chocolate.

Divide the ice cream into plastic containers or individual forms and let them stand in the freezer for at least 4–5 hours. The ice cream needs time to soften so take it out of the freezer about half an hour before use.

Variation: Instead of chocolate, use berries or vanilla-flavoured sugar in the ice cream. Real ground vanilla, which you can buy in health food shops, tastes best. If you mix 1 tsp real vanilla with 10 tsp erythritol, you get vanilla-flavoured sugar – but do experiment and find the combination that works best for you.

CHOCOLATE FROMAGE

Makes 4–6 portions

5 sheets of gelatine
3 eggs
5 tbs erythritol
2 tbs cacao
300 ml (10.5 fl oz) whipping cream

Put the gelatine sheets to soak in cold water for about 5 minutes. Then melt them in a small pot with about 5 tbs boiling water in the bottom.

Beat the eggs and 3 tbs erythritol together and fold the egg mixture into the gelatine (not the reverse).

Stir 2 tbs erythritol and cacao into the whipping cream and whip the cream until it is stiff.

Fold the whipped cream carefully into the egg mixture.

Put the whole thing in a suitable serving bowl and put it in the refrigerator, preferably overnight.

The fromage can be decorated with whipped cream, grated 70 % chocolate and sliced almonds.

CHOCOLATE MOUSSE

Makes 6–8 portions

150 g (5.25 oz) 70 % chocolate
2 tbs strong coffee
300 ml (10.5 fl oz) whipping cream
3 eggs, separated into yolks and whites
100 g (10.5 oz) erythritol

Melt the chocolate together with the coffee in a double-boiler.

Whip the cream until stiff.

In another bowl beat the egg yolks and erythritol until thick and fluffy.

Blend the chocolate mixture with the egg mixture.

Beat the egg whites stiff in a third bowl.

Blend the chocolate mixture with the whipped cream and, finally, fold in the beaten egg whites.

Put the mousse in a serving bowl or dessert dishes. Let it chill for at least two hours in the refrigerator before serving.

Garnish as you like with cream sweetened with erythritol or sliced almonds.

APPLE DESSERT

Makes 4–6 portions

4 apples
2 tbs erythritol
1 tsp cinnamon
20 chopped almonds

Divide the apples into quarters and distribute them in an oven-proof dish. Sprinkle on erythritol, cinnamon and chopped almonds.

Bake the apples in the middle of the oven at 200 °C (400 °F) for about 20 minutes, or until they are soft.

The apple dessert can be eaten as it is, or with whipped cream.

SORBET

Makes 1 portion

200 g (7 oz) frozen berries
1 small cup natural yogurt
1 tsp lemon juice
4 tbs erythritol

Mix all the ingredients with a hand blender or food processor, and the dessert is ready for serving.

CONFECTIONARY

250 g (8.75 oz) coconut fat
250 g (8.75 oz) 70 % chocolate
300–400 g (10.5 – 14 oz) chopped nuts or almonds

Melt the coconut fat.

Break the chocolate into pieces and melt them in a double-boiler.

Pour the melted coconut fat into the melted chocolate and mix well. Fill a suitable pan with chopped nuts or almonds. Then pour the chocolate mixture over the nuts. Cool the chocolate mixture in the fridge until it hardens.

Cut the chocolate into small pieces. Keep them cool or freeze them.

Variation: For a fresher taste, you can add the grated peel of 2 oranges.

CHEESE CRISPS

Grate a good white cheese or parmesan and form it into small peaks on baking paper on a baking sheet. Bake the cheese peaks in the middle of the oven at 175 °C (350 °F) for 4–5 minutes, or until they have turned a golden colour. Take care that they don't get burnt! You can make cheese crisps in the microwave oven as well. In this case, use a cheese slicer to make cheese slices, let them stand in the microwave oven until they bubble – which usually takes about 2 minutes. Let them cool. Cheese crisps taste good with soups, as snacks, and they can be used for tacos instead of tortillas or taco shells.

CHEESE PLATTER

Various cheeses
Various vegetables
Olives

If you want to put the cheese on something (instead of crackers or bread), try slices of cucumber or courgette (zucchini).

Glossary

Symbols

> = greater than
< = less than
≥ = greater than or equal

Blood test results

Blood test results

Reference range

When you receive results from blood tests, you usually get a value that relates specifically to you, and also a "reference range". This reference range has been made by examining a certain number of healthy people, of whom 95 % have values which lie within the reference range. The reference range can change over time, because the population changes. That means that the reference values do not necessarily reflect that which is optimal. In the case histories in this book, the reference range is given after the blood test result in question. For some blood test results, the reference ranges are different for women and men and different for different age groups. Different laboratories can also have different reference ranges because they may use slightly different methods for the measurements. I have myself defined C-peptide > 700 pmol/L and triglycerides > 1.7 mmol/L as excessive values. You will find my reason under C-peptide and triglycerides in this overview.

Blood sugar

A blood sugar measurement tells you how much glucose there is in your blood at the time the measurement was taken. A fasting blood sugar tells you how much glucose there is in your blood after a night's fasting. In Norway, a fasting blood sugar between 4 and 6 mmol/L is defined as normal. Fasting blood sugar over 6 mmol/L is defined as high and over 7 mmol/L as diabetes. The American Diabetes Association has defined a fasting blood sugar over 5.6 mmol/L as high, but the diabetes boundary has been set at 7 mmol/L, the same as in Norway. Excessive levels of sugar in the blood are lowered on a low carbohydrate diet. For people with type 1 diabetes, this assumes correct dosing of insulin.

Long-term blood sugar – HbA1c

HbA_{1c} is a marker for the level of glucose in the blood over a long period. Glucose binds itself to haemoglobin in the red blood cells, and the amount of glucose that is bound to haemoglobin says something about the concentration of glucose in the blood. The HbA_{1c} value reflects the average blood sugar over the last six-eight weeks. High values are, therefore, recorded when a patient has an increased average blood sugar. People with poorly-regulated diabetes often have higher levels of HbA_{1c} than usual. A person with diabetes and well-regulated blood sugar has a HbA_{1c} level near or within the normal range. In the following table you can see the connection between HbA_{1c} and average blood sugar.

The connection between HbA1c and average blood sugar.

HbA1c (%)	Average blood sugar (mmol/L)
5	4.5
6	6.7
7	8.3
8	10.0
9	11.6
10	13.3
11	15.0
12	16.7

As the table shows, a patient may have an extremely high average blood sugar when HbA_{1c} is 12 %. Fürst laboratorium in Oslo uses the reference range < 6.1 percent. That is to say, 95 % of the healthy Norwegian population has values under 6.1 percent. The treatment goal for diabetics in Norway has been set at < 7.0 percent. If you look at the table, you can see that a patient will have an average blood sugar of approximately 8.3 mmol/L if HbA_{1c} is 7.0 percent. Long-term blood sugar is lowered on a diet with few carbohydrates. For people with type 1 diabetes, this assumes correct dosing of insulin.

C-peptide and insulin

C-peptide is an expression for the production of insulin in the pancreas. When insulin is created, equal amounts of C-peptide and insulin are released from pro-insulin (an amino acid chain). C-peptide is broken down more slowly than insulin and is, therefore, a more reliable measure of insulin production than insulin. Among the great majority of people, insulin production is determined by the sugar level in the blood and increases with increasing insulin resistance.

I have defined C-peptide over 700 pmol/L (sample taken after fasting) as an expression for insulin resistance, because the upper reference value was 720 pmol/L at the Hormone Laboratory, Aker Hospital in Oslo before 2004, and the method that is used today is unchanged. The fact that the reference value has increased reflects an increasing insulin resistance in the population. Excessive values of C-peptide and insulin are lowered on a carbohydrate-restricted diet. Among patients who are being treated with insulin, C-peptide can be used to assess the patient's own production of insulin.

Triglycerides

Triglycerides are fats. After a high fat meal, we have a lot of triglycerides in the blood, and this fat will be used for various tasks in the body. Triglycerides are broken down into fatty acids, which are used as fuel by the muscles. By taking a blood sample, triglycerides can be measured after a night's fast. Various diseases can yield high triglyceride values, but it is most common with a high consumption of sugar and starch. If you eat more carbohydrates than you have use for, triglycerides are formed from glucose. This process also occurs at night. You can, therefore, have a high fasting triglyceride level if you eat a lot of carbohydrates. When the consumption of carbohydrates is reduced significantly, the triglyceride level is generally lowered. Having lots of triglycerides does not result in symptoms except at extremely high values, but it is still considered a contributory factor for developing cardiovascular disease. I have set the reference range for triglycerides at less than 1.7 mmol/L, as values over 1.7 mmol/L are used as one of the criteria for metabolic syndrome, while the reference range at the laboratories has been set at < 2.60 mmol/L.

Total cholesterol

In established scientific environments, it's thought that there is a clear connection between total cholesterol and the risk for developing vascular disease in the heart. For that reason, cholesterol-lowering medication is used in the event of excessive levels. Less than 5 mmol/L is usually considered to be a desirable level for total cholesterol, 5–6.4 mmol/L is called slightly elevated; 6.5–7.9 mmol/L moderately elevated; while over 8 mmol/L is defined as extremely high total cholesterol. More recent studies have shown that a patient's total cholesterol value is lowered on a low carb diet. Clinical experience shows that the level of total cholesterol generally goes down with the consumption of few carbohydrates and a lot of fat, but with some people the cholesterol value is unchanged. A very few get elevated values after starting a low carb diet, especially with high consumption of milk fat.

Traditionally, the focus is on the molecules the blood uses to transport cholesterol, namely the lipoproteins. They are classified according to density and are found in several varieties. The most discussed are LDL and HDL.

LDL cholesterol

The LDL molecule transports cholesterol out to the cells. LDL cholesterol has been called "the bad cholesterol" because it's thought that a high level is particularly unhealthy. The LDL cholesterol value generally decreases on a low carb diet. The LDL molecules can have various qualities – some are large and "airy", while others are small and dense. Most experts believe that the large, "airy" LDL molecules are not dangerous, in contrast to the small, dense ones.

HDL cholesterol

HDL molecules transport used cholesterol from cells to the liver. The HDL cholesterol is called "the good cholesterol" because it's thought that a high level protects against cardiovascular disease. Overweight people who eat a lot of high carb foods often have low HDL cholesterol values, at the same time as they have high levels of triglycerides. When carbohydrate consumption is reduced, the triglyceride value generally goes down and the HDL cholesterol value goes up. This is a more favourable profile with a view to cardiovascular disease.

Homocysteine

Homocysteine is an amino acid – one of the building blocks of proteins. It is produced in our body and works in interaction with folate, vitamin B12 and vitamin B6. Supplements of these vitamins generally reduce the homocysteine level if there is a deficiency of them at the outset. Homocysteine is a recognised contributor to cardiovascular diseases. However, it has not been shown that a reduction of the homocysteine level with B vitamins lowers the incidence of such diseases. So long as we know that an elevated level is associated with a risk for disease, I consider a lower level to be desirable. My experience is that a low carb diet consisting of mostly natural foods reduces homocysteine levels.

Micro-CRP

CRP stands for C-reactive protein. Laboratories have a method for measuring extremely low values of CRP, that is

Micro-CRP. CRP is produced in the liver when you have an inflammation in your body. It is one of several substances the body makes to fight against infections and inflammations. These substances set in motion several reactions. It isn't known with certainty what functions the protein has, but it is known that it takes part in this process, and that it can be used as a measure of how strong an infection or inflammation is. The reference range for Micro-CRP is < 5 mg/L. A micro-CRP level over 4–5 mg/L is considered a contributory factor to developing cardiovascular disease, and many doctors now believe that inflammation is the most important cause for such diseases. Micro-CRP is often elevated in the case of insulin resistance and obesity. From experience, Micro-CRP is lowered when patients lose weight on a low carb diet.

Ferritin

Healthy adults have 3–4 g of iron in the body, and 60–70 % of this is found in the haemoglobin in the red blood cells. The remainder is stored in the liver, the spleen and in bone marrow. The iron is bound to special proteins, and the most common is called ferritin, which is a good measure of the general level of iron in the body. The ferritin level is often measured in order to investigate whether the patient has an iron deficiency or haemochromatosis. Haemochromatosis is a genetic disease that causes iron to pile up in the body, because it isn't being excreted in step with the intake.

Ferritin belongs to a class of proteins that are called acute phase proteins, which means proteins that are released in large amounts in the blood in the event of infection and inflammation. If you have an acute infection or chronic inflammation in your body, you may have high values of ferritin without necessarily having a lot of iron stored in your body. If your insulin level is high, you probably have an inflammation somewhere in your body. Many people with insulin resistance and type 2 diabetes have high ferritin levels. The ferritin value is generally normalised when the insulin level is lowered.

ALAT and gamma GT

ALAT and gamma GT are enzymes found especially in the liver. If the liver is overburdened or is damaged, these enzymes leak out of the cells and are found in the blood in larger amounts than is normal. Doctors who examine the liver with ultrasound see fatty livers more and more often with obesity. Accumulation of fat can be the reason that these liver enzymes are very often elevated in the blood of overweight people. However, they normalise with weight loss when obesity is the cause.

Creatinine

Creatinine is a measure of kidney function. High values are seen with kidney failure. My experience is that creatinine values that are slightly too high are generally lowered on a low carb diet.

Uric acid

Uric acid is a substance which is formed in the body when purines are broken down. Purines are important constituents in the body's cells. Foods with high purine content include: meat, offal, seafood, yeast, alcoholic beverages, pulses, rolled oats, spinach, asparagus, cauliflower and mushrooms. Uric acid has no important function in the body, and the surplus is therefore excreted via the kidneys.

Patients with gout have too much uric acid in the blood, and in more than 90 % of cases, it's because the kidneys are not excreting the substance effectively enough. The traditional treatment is to reduce the consumption of purines in the diet. Anti-inflammatory medications are given for the intense pain.

Patients can take preventive medication to reduce the level of uric acid in the blood, but, more importantly, insulin reduces the excretion of uric acid in the kidneys, so that the amount in the blood increases. A great many of my patients have too much uric acid in their blood. The level is normalised on a low carb diet, even if they eat quantities of purine-containing meat.

TSH

TSH is an abbreviation for the thyroid-stimulating hormone, which is produced in the pituitary gland in the brain. TSH stimulates the thyroid gland to produce the metabolic hormones thyroxine (T_4) and triiodothyronine (T_3). The TSH level is usually high with hypothyroidism (low metabolism) and low with hyperthyroidism (high metabolism). TSH is used to monitor treatment with thyroxine, which is given in the case of hypothyroidism. From experience, excessive levels of TSH are often lowered when a person eats natural low carb foods.

FT_4

FT_4 is an abbreviation for free thyroxine in the blood; it is a metabolic hormone. All the thyroxine circulating in the blood is produced in the thyroid gland. The FT_4 level is high with hyperthyroidism (high metabolism) and low with hypothyroidism (low metabolism).

FT₃

FT$_3$ is an abbreviation for free triiodothyronine; it is a metabolic hormone. Ten to twenty percent of all triiodothyronine in the blood is produced in the thyroid gland, while the remainder is created in the liver and kidneys from thyroxine. Triiodothyronine is five to six times more active than thyroxine. The value can increase before FT$_4$ does in an early phase of high metabolism. A low value can mean that the transformation of FT$_4$ to FT$_3$ is not functioning as it should.

Anti-TPO

Anti-TPOs are antibodies which attack and can damage the thyroid gland. A high anti-TPO level can over time lead to hypothyroidism (low metabolism). I have seen several times that anti-TPOs are reduced on a low carb diet.

Testosterone

Testosterone is a so-called "androgenic" – or "growth-promoting" – hormone which is produced in the testicles of men, in the ovaries of women and in the adrenal cortex in both men and women. It is the dominant sex hormone in men and stimulates development of male characteristics such as the growth of the sex organs and the larynx. Testosterone promotes voice change during puberty, the growth of increased muscle mass, of a beard and body hair, and it is important for sexual function and erection. Testosterone circulates freely in the blood and is bound to the sexual hormone binding globulin (SHBG). Several studies have shown a connection between metabolic syndrome and low testosterone levels in men. The testosterone level is generally normalised if they lose weight.

If the testosterone level is too high among women, menstruation can become irregular or not occur at all. In addition, there is more obvious hair growth, especially where it's typical for men. My experience is that the testosterone level usually goes down when women switch to a low carb diet.

SHBG – sexual hormone binding globulin

SHBG is produced in the liver. Its production and concentration in the blood increases under the influence of oestrogen and decreases with testosterone. Low values are often seen in women who have too much testosterone, and high values when women use oestrogen and during pregnancy. In men, low values are seen with the use of anabolic steroids and high levels of testosterones, but levels are high with low testosterone production or increased oestrogen production. Experience shows that SHBG often normalises when insulin levels normalise on a low carb diet.

Selenium

Selenium is part of a number of enzyme systems and is important for our health. A low intake of selenium has been linked with an increased risk for cancer. Several studies have shown that selenium supplements can reduce the risk for certain types of cancer. Selenium strengthens the immune system, and protects against heavy metal toxins. Good sources of selenium are Brazil nuts, meat, fish, shellfish, milk, cheese and eggs. Two Brazil nuts covers the daily requirement.

Zinc

Zinc is a cofactor in at least 200 of the body's enzymes, which are part of the body's tools for converting carbohydrates, proteins and fat. Zinc is important for the function of DNA, for formation and growth of tissues and organs, for the healing of wounds, the immune system, sense of taste, hormone production and brain function. Good sources for zinc are beef, offal, shellfish, chicken, fish, eggs, whole grains and nuts. Zinc from plant sources such as grain are not absorbed as easily from the intestine as zinc from animal products.

Magnesium

Magnesium is part of over 300 different enzyme systems in the body. It has a central role in the body's metabolism, and insufficient magnesium leads to a reduced insulin effect. Magnesium stabilises the heart's rhythm, is important for maintaining normal blood pressure and for the muscles functioning as they should. Good sources of magnesium are vegetables, nuts, almonds, seeds, meat, poultry, fish, shellfish, seafood and whole grains.

Vitamin D

This is a fat-soluble vitamin which cannot be excreted in the urine. Consumption of extremely large doses of vitamin D can theoretically accumulate in the body and be toxic, but vitamin D poisoning is extremely rare. A lack of vitamin D is more common and can lead to damage to the skeleton. There are few foods which contribute significant amounts of vitamin D. Oily fish, fish liver and cod liver oil have a high content, and other important sources are butter and egg yolks. In the summer we produce vitamin D when we are out in the sunshine. A relatively large portion of the population has unsatisfactory levels of vitamin D in the blood (under 50 nmol/L), and there is a higher incidence in winter. Half an hour of summer sun on the body provides us a lot of vitamin D. Ten minutes daily of sun on the face and arms is enough to get a good production of vitamin D, if you get it every day in the summer. During the winter, it can be beneficial to have a ten minute session in a solarium twice a week or to take a supplement. People with dark skin need more sun than people with white skin in order to produce enough vitamin D.

This vitamin is the subject of much research, and several studies show that a good store of vitamin D in the body prevents cancer. People who are overweight and have insulin resistance and diabetes have especially low levels of vitamin D, but we still don't know exactly why. According to international researchers, the level in the blood should lie somewhere between 100–150 nmol/L.

Vitamin B_{12}

This vitamin is important for normal nerve function and the formation of blood cells. Foods from animals or insects are the only dietary sources for vitamin B_{12}. Most people have a store of vitamin B_{12} in the body, so that it can take many years before a deficiency arises. Vitamin B_{12} deficiency can lead to anaemia, nerve damage and mental illness. It may be due to insufficient consumption or insufficient uptake of vitamin B_{12}. Vegans should take a vitamin B_{12} supplement. Vegetarians who don't eat meat and few dairy products should have their blood checked and possibly take a supplement.

Folate

Folate is a water-soluble B-vitamin which is found in nearly all foods. The amount of folate is especially high in green vegetables, liver and pulses. Illness caused by folate deficiency is rare, but too little folate in the diet can result in anaemia. Studies have shown that increasing folate consumption can reduce the risk of cardiovascular disease and several types of cancer. Pregnant and lactating women require considerable amounts of folate, and a deficiency can lead to serious damage to the foetus, such as spina bifida and cleft palates. All women who plan to become pregnant are advised to take a folate supplement.

Other medical expressions

Insulin

Insulin is a hormone which is created in the pancreas and is secreted into the blood in order to transport sugar from the blood into the cells. The hormone is secreted in different amounts depending on food consumption and blood sugar level. Too little production of insulin or deficient effect from insulin (insulin resistance) leads to excessive blood sugar levels. Too much insulin leads to low blood sugar (hypoglycaemia). Insulin also functions as a tissue-building hormone in protein and fat metabolism. That's why high levels of insulin in the blood lead to weight gain.

Insulin resistance

Insulin resistance is a condition wherein the cells in the body have become less sensitive to insulin because they don't want to absorb more glucose. In order to compensate for this, the pancreas produces more insulin. The muscle and liver cells become insulin resistant before fatty tissue does. This results in the fat cells taking up more glucose and converting it to fat. When the fat cells refuse to accept surplus glucose from the bloodstream, the blood sugar rises and the patient develops type 2 diabetes. The principal cause of insulin resistance is that more carbohydrates are being consumed than the body has use for.

Cortisol

This vital hormone is a steroid hormone, which is to say that it is made via conversion of cholesterol. It has an important role in calming the immune response, but it also functions as a "stress hormone". Cortisol is produced in the adrenal glands and can be confirmed in blood and saliva. The level increases with mental and physical stress and when the blood sugar level is too low, as is the case with glucagon, adrenalin and growth hormone. The evolutionary explanation for this is that we have developed several safety mechanisms to counteract low blood sugar (but only one to counteract high blood sugar: insulin).

When you're stressed, you're more exposed to infections than when you are mentally relaxed, because the increased cortisol level inhibits the immune system. With chronic stress, you have a chronically elevated cortisol level, which leads to increased fat on the belly and the neck, and, in some cases, more body hair. This occurs because cortisol breaks down body proteins, including connective tissue, and converts it to glucose. Because of the breaking down of protein, a high cortisol level can result in stretch marks, even in men.

Cortisone

Cortisone is a synthetic pharmaceutical with a similar effect to cortisol. Cortisone is often used to suppress the immune system in diseases such as asthma, eczema and rheumatic disorders. Many people notice that they put on weight when they take cortisone. The explanation is described under cortisol.

Metabolic syndrome

Insulin resistance is believed to be the principal cause for what is called metabolic syndrome or syndrome X, which is a collective term for several adverse effects of a chronically elevated insulin level. Among other things, it increases the risk for cardiovascular disease, overweight, increase belly fat, fats in the blood, elevated blood pressure and the inability to maintain normal blood sugar levels. The criteria for metabolic syndrome, according to the International Diabetes Federation, are:

- Waist measurement for men > 94 centimetres (37 inches) and for women > 80 centimetres (31.5 inches). In addition to an increased waist measurement, the patient must have at least two of the following four risk factors:
- Triglycerides > 1.7 mmol/L, or being treated for high triglyceride level
- HDL cholesterol < 0.9 mmol/L for men and < 1.1 mmol/L for women, or being treated for low HDL cholesterol level
- Blood pressure with systolic > 130 or diastolic > 85, or being treated for high blood pressure
- Fasting blood sugar > 5.6 mmol/L, or diabetes

Autoimmune diseases

Autoimmune diseases are a group of diseases in which the immune system interprets components in the patient's own body as foreign. The body therefore attacks its own cells and tissues. These attacks can lead to diseases such as low metabolism, type 1 diabetes, arthritis and connective tissue disease.

Overview of carbohydrate content in foods

This overview shows how many grams of carbohydrates there are in 100 grams of a food product. The lists are organised from low to high content. If you need more detailed information search online for "nutritional value".

Vegetables	Carbohydrates
Leaf lettuce	0.3
Mushrooms	0.3
Spinach	0.4
Avocado	0.5
Spinach, frozen	0.5
Head lettuce	0.7
Cabbage	0.9
Endive	1.0
Asparagus	1.1
Cucumber	1.2
Chive	1.3
Celery stalk	1.3
Artichoke	1.3
Iceberg lettuce	1.5
Parsley	1.6
Chinese cabbage	1.8
Broccoli	1.9
Kale	2.2

Vegetables	Carbohydrates
Courgette (zucchini)	2.2
Aubergine	2.2
Cauliflower	2.3
Radish	2.5
Tomato	2.5
Celery root	2.8
Pumpkin	2.8
Kohlrabi	3.0
Sweet green pepper	3.3
Red cabbage	3.4
Green beans, fresh	3.4
Leek	3.6
Brussels sprouts, frozen	4.3
Sweet yellow pepper	4.4
Brussels sprouts, fresh	4.4
Sweet red pepper	4.6
Turnip	4.7
Head cabbage	5.2

Vegetables

Sugar peas	5.3
Onion	5.7
Swede (Rutabaga)	6.4
Carrot	6.7
Parsley root	7.3
Peas, frozen	8.0
Beetroot	8.9
Parsnip	10.1
Sweet corn, fresh	12.6
Garlic	16.3

Vegetables products

Olives, green	0.3
(Common) mushroom, tinned	0.7
Asparagus, tinned	1.7
Olives, black	1.8
Tomato, tinned	3.0
Tomato juice	3.0
Sauerkraut	5.1
Cucumbers, pickled	6.1
Tomato purée	12.9
Beetroot, pickled	13.6
Sweet corn, tinned	16.5
Tomato ketchup	23.5
Chestnuts, roasted	36.6

Pulses

Beans in tomato sauce	14.3
Peas, dried	16.2
Beans, brown cooked	17.4
Soybeans, dried	18.9
Mung beans, dried	38.3
Peas, yellow, dried	41.4
Beans, white, dried	41.4
Chickpeas, dried	42.0
Beans, brown, dried	44.6

Potatoes

New potatoes	11.2
Mashed potato, powder, milk	13.6
Potatoes, tinned	15.1
Potatoes, fall harvest	15.3
Potatoes, storage potatoes	16.6
Oven-baked chips	22.0
Chips, deep fried	39.8

Fruit, fresh

Avocado	0.5
Rhubarb	0.7
Lime	0.8
Lemon	2.2
Melon, cantaloupe	4.2
Melon, honeydew	5.6
Passion fruit	5.8
Grapefruit	6.8
Apricot	7.2
Orange	7.2
Melon, watermelon	7.6
Peach	7.6
Pomegranate	7.8
Pear	8.0
Clementine	8.7
Papaya	8.8
Nectarine	9.0
Plum	9.3
Apple	10.0
Pineapple	10.1
Kiwi fruit	10.6
Grape, red	11.7
Mango	14.1
Grape, green	16.0
Banana	18.1

Berries, fresh

Raspberries	3.2
Cloudberries	4.4
Gooseberries	5.4
Blackberries	6.4
Strawberries	6.6
Redcurrants	6.9
Lingonberries	7.0
Elderberries	7.4
Blueberries	7.5
Blackcurrant	7.6
Cherries	9.0
Morello cherries	11.2

Dried fruit

Prunes	36.5
Apricot	43.4
Figs	53.9
Apple	57.2
Raisins	65.8
Dates	68.0

Tinned fruit

Fruit cocktail, own juice	7.2
Pear, own juice	8.5
Peach, own juice	9.7
Pineapple, own juice	12.2
Pear, in syrup	13.2
Peach, in syrup	14.0
Fruit cocktail, in syrup	14.8
Plum, in syrup	15.5
Apricot, in syrup	16.1
Pineapple, in syrup	16.5

Nuts and almonds

Brazil nuts	3.1
Walnuts	3.3
Pecans	5.8
Hazel nuts	6.0
Almonds	6.9
Peanuts, salted	7.7
Pistachio nuts, salted	8.2
Peanuts, unsalted	12
Cashew nuts, unsalted	18.1

Milk and dairy products

Normal white cheese	0
Mozzarella	1.0
Feta cheese	1.5
Cottage cheese	1.5
Whole fat sour cream, 35 %	1.6
Créme fraîche	1.6
Whipping cream, 38 %	2.6
Chevre goat cheese	3.0
Cream cheese	3.0
Philadelphia cream cheese, original	3.2
Low fat sour cream, 20 %	3.2
Parmesan	3.7
Cooking cream, 22 %	3.8
Fermented milk	4.0
Coffee cream, 10 %	4.2
Whole fat milk	4.6
Semi skimmed milk	4.7
Quark	4.8
Natural yogurt	5.5
Activia pouring yogurt, strawberry	7.3
Activia yogurt, raspberry	11.0
Fruit yogurt (0.1 %)	12.2
Fruit yogurt (0.5 %)	12.4
Ice cream	23.0
Frozen yogurt	29.0
Coffee-mate powder	57.3

Meat, eggs and fish

Pure meat	0
Fish	0

296

Caviar, from capelin   0
Eggs 0.3
Liver pâté, tinned 1.8
Meat balls, tinned 1.9
Salami, sheep 2.1
Patty, ox, fried 2.9
Meat cakes 3.7
Sausage, low fat 4.0
Fish pâté, salmon 4.3
Sausage, chicken 4.9
Medister 4.9
Bologna sausage 5.0
Meat sausage 5.0
Mackerell in tomato,
tinned 5.2
Fish balls, refrigerated
product 5.2
Fish patties, lean fish 5.3
Wiener sausage, sport
wiener 5.3
Sausage 5.4
Meatloaf, cooked 6.2
Fish balls, tinned 6.6
Saithe steak, breaded,
with onion 6.7
Fish pudding 7.1
Fish cakes 8.0
Crabsticks, frozen 10.7
Anchovies, tinned 12.1
Caviar, from cod 13.7
Fish gratin without eggs,
frozen 14.7
Fish sticks, deep fried,
frozen 17.4
Cod, deep fried, frozen 17.4
Pickled herring, drained . . . 20.8
Blood pudding 24.3
Spiced pickled herring 24.5
Mustard herring 25.6

Flour

Soybean meal 23.5
Flour, wholemeal 54.4
Flour, sifted 63.9

Grain, rice, pasta

Pasta, green, fresh 54.2
Pasta naturelle, fresh, raw . . 56.3
Rolled oats 63.1
Pasta naturelle, dry 69.8
Rice, polished, long-grain,
dry 75.9
Rice, polished, basmati
rice, dry 76.8
Rice, polished, jasmine
rice, dry 79.5
Porridge rice, dry 80.5

Cereal

All Bran plus 47.4
4-grain 59.2
Shredded oats 63.0
Weetabix 67.4
Puffed oats 69.1
Cornflakes 81.6
Honey oats 82.5
Puffed rice 85.4

Cooked grain, rice, pasta

Pasta naturelle, fresh 18.2
Pasta, green, fresh 19.3
Nature rice, long-grain 19.5
Minute rice 20.8
Polished, long-grain rice . . . 26.4
Spaghetti/macaroni 26.5
Bulgur 27.7
Wheat noodles, no eggs 27.7
Couscous 28.6

Homebaked bread products

Bread, 100 % wholemeal, water	37.6
Gluten-free, wholemeal, milk	40.3
Bread, 50 % wholemeal, water	40.9
French bread, milk	45.5
Gluten-free, flour, milk	46.3

Industry baked bread products

Potato cake, lefse, potato	39.3
Pumpernickel	37.0
Rye bread, wholemeal	38.7
Norwegian mountain bread	39.9
Four-grain bread	40.4
Wholemeal bread, no syrup	41.2
Wholemeal bread, with syrup	41.4
Birkebeiner bread	42.4
Pita bread, fine	42.7
Rye bread, fine	45.7
Tortilla, corn	46.2
French bread, white bread	46.6
Rolls, fine	47.4
Hamburger buns, fine	49.2
Baguettes, fine	50.6
Hotdog buns, fine	51.4

Crisp bread, crackers

Bran bread, with wheat bran	38.5
Crisp bread, extra fiber	43.2
Tacoshells	56.0
Crisp bread, rye, wholemeal	62.0

Baked goods, cakes

Sandwich biscuits, oat biscuits	63.5
Crisp bread, rye	63.7
Flat bread, homemade type	65.5
Crisp bread, white	67.7
Crisp bread, gluten-free	71.1
Rice cakes	78.0

Cookies, biscuits

Ring cake	52.8
Cookies	60.7
Crackers, sweet, wholemeal	62.9
Crackers, sweet, filled	68.9
Crackers, sweet, children's crackers	74.8

Baked goods, cakes

Cream puffs, no filling	20.2
Cheesecake with biscuit base	24.8
Waffles with eggs, whole fat milk	24.8
Sponge cake, whipped cream, jam	29.4
Pastry, egg cream	35.9
Nut base	36.8
Carrot cake	42.3
Wheat bun with whole fat milk	45.9
Prince's cake, almonds	47.0
Chocolate cake with frosting	47.2
Gluten-free buns	48.3

Sugar and sweets

Snowballs 30.9
Marzipan 47.7
Milk chocolate 53.1
Chocolate spread 57.8
Chocolate, filled 60.2
Nut spread 65.2
Honey 67.0
Hard candy, filled 68.6
Licorice candy 68.7
Syrup 76.6
Jelly Babies 79.7

Chewing gum with sugar ... 81.0
Assorted candies,
no chocolate 88.5
Sugar, brown sugar,
powdered sugar 100

Miscellaneous

Bacon crisps 0.1
Cheese doodles 44.0
Popcorn, bought 51.7
Potato crisps 54.7
Tortilla crisps 56.0

Drinks, ready to drink

Tea, black 0
Coffee 0
Orange squash 8.4
Chocolate milk 9.0
Blackurrant syrup/
squash 9.5
Soda 10.0
Orange juice 10.0
Apple nectar 10.2
Squash 10.4
Milkshake, strawberry
flavour 11.0
Grape juice 11.1
Hot cocoa, instant 13.0

Beer, wine and spirits

Spirits, 60 % 0
White wine, dry, 12 % 0.2
Red wine, 12 % 0.8
Spirits, 40 % 2.0
Light beer, 2.5 % 2.5
White wine, medium
dry, 10 % 2.9
Lager, 4.7 % 3.2
Alcohol-free beer 3.4
Fortified wine,
sweet, 17 % 10.0

Recipe index

Bibliography

English language, with references to scientific literature

Allan CB, Lutz W. Life Without Bread: How A Low Carb Diet Can Save Your Life. California: Keats Publishing, 2000.

Atkins RC. Dr. Atkins' New Diet Revolution. New York: HarperCollins Publishers, 2001.

Cleave TL. The saccharine disease. New Canaan: Keats Publishing, 1975.

Cordain L. The paleo diet. New York: John Wiley & Sons, 2002.

Enig MG. Know your fats. Silver Spring: Bethesda Press, 2008.

Groves B. Trick and treat. London: Hammersmith Press, 2008.

Kabara JJ. Fats are good for you and other secrets. Berkeley: North Atlantic Books, 2008.

Kendrick M. The Great Cholesterol Con: The Truth About What Really Causes Heart Disease and How to Avoid It. London: John Blake Publishing Ltd, 2007.

McDonald L. The ketogenic diet. A complete guide for the dieter and practitioner. Austin Tx: Morris Publishing, 1998.

Mercola J, Levy AR. The no-grain diet. London: Hodder and Stoughton, 2005.

Ravnskov U. Fat and Cholesterol Are GOOD for You. Sweden: GB Publishing, 2009.

Rosedale R, Colman C. The Rosedale diet. New York: HarperCollins Publishers, 2004.

Starr M. Hypothyroidism type 2. The epidemic. Colombia, MO: Mark Starr Trust, 2005, 2007.

Su RK. Carbohydrates can kill. Minneapolis: Two Harbors Press, 2009.

Taubes G. Good calories, bad calories. New York: Alfred A Knopf, 2007.

**English language,
without references to scientific literature**
Enig M, Fallon S. Eat fat, loose fat. London: Penguin books, 2005.

Groves B. Natural health and weight loss. London: Hammersmith Press, 2007.

Kwasniewski J. Optimal nutrition. Warszawa: Wydawnictwo WPG, 1999. Bought at www.wgp.com.pl.

Litsfeldt LE. Diabetes? No Thanks! The Scandinavian Diet that alleviates diabetes. Oslo: Little Moon Publishing, 2011.

Skaldeman SS. Lose Weight by Eating: The Scandinavian Diet. Oslo: Little Moon Publishing, 2011.

English language, academic books
Boron FB, Boulpaep EL. Medical physiology. Philadelphia: Saunders Elsevier, 2009.

**Nordic languages, not available in English,
with references to scientific literature**
Andersen TP. Slank med ketolysekuren. En enklere vei til et lettere liv. Oslo: Gyldendal, 2005.

Andersen TP. Etter slankekuren. Oslo: Gyldendal, 2005.

Erlanson-Albertsson C. Socker och fett på gott och ont. Västerås: ICA Bokförlag, 2004.

Clayton P. Helseguiden. Oslo: Press, 2005

Dahlqvist, A. Doktor Dahlqvists guide til LCHF. Et revolusjonerende kosthold for optimal helse. Oslo: Lille Måne, 2009.

Johnsson B, Nordström P. Sukkerbomben. Bli kvitt søtsuget. Oslo: Aschehoug, 2005.

Lindberg FA. Naturlig slank med kost i balanse. Oslo: Gyldendal, 2001.

Lindberg FA. Fedons metode. Naturlig slank med Kost i balanse. Oslo: Gyldendal, 2006.

Lindberg FA, Hansen-Møllerud M. Barn i balanse. Oslo: Gyldendal, 2008.

Lindeberg S. Mat – bedre helse med steinalderkost. Oslo: Humanist forlag AS, 2005.

Mysterud I. Mat, menneske og evolusjon. Oslo: Gyldendal Akademisk, 2006.

Nilssson F. Istället för doping. Sundbyberg: Pagina Förlags AB/Optimal Förlag, 2009.

Paulún F. Alt om fettforbrenning. Oslo: Cappelen Damm, 2002.

Paulún F. Blodsockerblues – en bok om glykemiskt index. Stockholm: Fitnessförlaget, 2002.

Poleszynski DV. Kostkontroll mot sukkersyke og overvekt. Oslo: Baibooks AS, 2008.

Poleszynski DV, Mysterud I. Sukker – en snikende fare. Oslo: Gyldendal Akademisk, 2004.

Sears B, Lawren B. Finn din sone. Oslo: Hilt & Hansteen AS, 2000.

Sears B. Hold deg ung i sonen. Oslo: Hilt & Hansteen AS, 2001.

Sears B. Omega-sonen. Oslo: Hilt & Hansteen AS, 2002.

Willett WC. Hold deg frisk med riktig kosthold. Oslo: Gyldendal,

Nordic languages, not available in English, based on personal experience

Bernstein, RK. Løsningen på diabetes. Oslo: Wem3 AS, 1997.

Litsfeldt LE. Spis deg sukkerfri. Oslo: Lille Måne, 2007.

Skaldeman SS. GI-null! Oslo: Lille Måne, 2008.

Skaldeman SS. Sten Sture Skaldemans kokebok. Oslo: Lille Måne, 2009.

Nordic languages, not available in English, academic books
Sand O, Sjaastad ØV, Haug E. Menneskets fysiologi. Oslo:
Gyldendal Akademisk, 2001.

Scientific articles
Abdullah AR, Hasan HA, Raigangar VL. Analysis of the
relationship of leptin, high-sensitivity C-reactive protein,
adiponectin, insulin, and uric acid to metabolic syndrome in
lean, overweight, and obese young females. Metab Syndr
Relat Disord 2009; 7: 17–22.

Accurso A, Bernstein RK, Dahlqvist A et al. Dietary
carbohydrate restriction in type 2 diabetes mellitus and
metabolic syndrome: Time for a critical appraisal.
http://www.nutritionandmetabolism.com/ content/5/1/9.

Anderson JW, Kendall CWC, Jenkins DJA. Importance of weight
management in type 2 diabetes: Review with meta-analysis of
clinical studies. J Am Coll Nutr 2003; 22: 331–9.

Angelillo VA, Bedi S, Durfee D et al. Effects of low and high
carbohydrate feedings in ambulatory patients with chronic
obstructive pulmonary disease and chronic hypercapnia. Ann
Intern Med 1985; 103: 883–5.

Aronson D, Rayfield EJ. How hyperglycemia promotes
atherosclerosis: Molecular mechanisms.
http://www.cardiab.com/content/1/1/1.

Arora SK, McFarlane SI. The case for low carbohydrate diets in
diabetes management.
http://www.nutritionandmetabolism.com/content/2/1/16.

Azadbakht L, Mirmiran P, Esmaillzadeh A et al. Dairy
consumption is inversely associated with the prevalence of
the metabolic syndrome in Tehranian adults. Am J Clin Nutr
2005; 82: 523–30.

Bacon CG, Hu FB, Giovannucci E et al. Association of type and
duration of diabetes with erectile dysfunction in a large
cohort of men. Diabetes Care 2002; 25: 1458–63.

Ball SD, Keller KR, Moyer-Mileur LJ et al. Prolongation of satiety after low versus moderately high glycemic index meals in obese adolescents. Pediatrics 2003; 111: 488–94.

Basciano H, Federico L, Adeli K. Fructose, insulin resistance, and metabolic dyslipidemia. http://www.nutritionandmetabolism.com/content/2/1/5.

Bassøe HH, Seim SH og Whitford M. Fettrik avmagringskost. Tidsskr Nor Lægeforen 1978, 98: 957-60.

Ben-Haroush A, Yogev Y, Hod M. Epidemiology of gestational diabetes mellitus and its association with type 2 diabetes. Diabetes Med 2004; 2: 103–13.

Biong AS, Rebnord HM, Fimreite RL et al. Intake of dairy fat and dairy products, and risk of myocardial infarction: A case-control study. Int J food Sci Nutr 2008; 59: 155–65.

Bloch AS. Low carbohydrate diets, pro: Time to rethink our current strategies. Nutr Clin Pract 2005; 20: 3–12.

Boden G, Sargrad K, Homko C. Effect of a low-carbohydrate diet on appetite, blood glucose levels, and insulin resistance in obese patients with type 2 diabetes. Ann Intern Med 2005; 142: 403–11.

Bouché C, Rizkalla SW, Jing L et al. Five-week, low-glycemic index diet decreases total fat mass and improves plasma lipid profile in moderately overweight nondiabetic men. Diabetes Care 2002; 25: 822-8.

Brehm BJ, Seeley RJ, Daniels SR et al. A randomized trial comparing a very low carbohydrate diet and a calorie-restricted low fat diet on body weight and cardiovascular risk factors in healthy women. J Clin Endocrinol Metab 2003; 88: 1617–23.

Capstick F, Brooks BA, Burns CM et al. Very low calorie diet (VLCD): A useful alternative in the treatment of the obese NIDDM patients. Diabetes Res Clin Pract 1997; 36: 105–11.

Carpenter MW. Gestational diabetes, pregnancy hypertension, and late vascular disease. Diabetes Care 2007; 30: S246–50.

Cavestro C, Rosatello A, Micca G et al. Insulin metabolism is altered in migraineurs: A new pathogenic mechanism for migraine? Headache 2007; 47: 1436-42.

Chen Z, Chen L, Dai H et al. Relationship between aminotranferase levels and metabolic syndrome in nonalcoholic fatty liver disease. J Zhejiang Univ Sci B 2008; 9: 616-22.

Choi HK, Willett CW, Stampfer MJ et al. Dairy consumption and risk of type 2 diabetes mellitus in men. Arch Intern Med 2005; 165: 997-1003.

Damm P. Gestational diabetes mellitus and subsequent development of overt diabetes mellitus. Dan Med Bull 1998; 45:495-509.

Dashti HM, Thazhumpal CM, Khadada M et al. Beneficial effects of ketogenic diet in obese diabetic subjects. Mol Cell Biochem 2007; 302: 249-56.

Del Prato S, Leonetti F, Simonson DC et al. Effect of sustained physiologic hyperinsulinaemia and hyperglycaemia on insulin secretion and insulin sensitivity in man. Diabetologia 1994; 37: 1025-35.

Dessein PH, Shipton EA, Stanwix AE et al. Beneficial effects of weight loss associated with moderate calorie/carbohydrate restriction, and increased proportional intake of protein and unsaturated fat on serum urate and lipoprotein levels in gout: A pilot study. Ann Rheum Dis 2000; 59: 539-43.

Dunlap BS, Bailes Jr JR. Unlimited energy, restricted carbohydrate diet improves lipid parameters in obese children. Metab Synd Relat Disord 2008; 6: 32-6.

Ebringer A, Wilson C. The use of a low starch diet in the treatment og patients suffering from ankylosing spondylitis. Clin Rhematol 1996; 15 Suppl 1: 62-6.

Eizirik DL, Korbutt GS, Hellerström C. Prolonged exposure of human pancreatic islets to high glucose concentrations in vitro impairs the ß-cell function. J Clin Invest 1992; 90: 1263-8.

Eriksson Susanne. Studies on nutrition, bone mineralization and metabolic markers in healthy 8-yr-olds in an urban swedish community. http://hdl/handle.net/2077/20457.

Esposito K, Nappo F, Marfella R et al. Inflammatory cytokine concentrations are acutely increased by hyperglycemia in humans: Role of oxidative stress. Circulation 2002; 106: 2067–72.

Farquhar JW, Frank A, Gross RC et al. Glucose, insulin, and triglyceride responses to high and low carbohydrate diets in man. J Clin Invest 1966; 45: 1648–56.

Feinman RD. When is a high fat diet not a high fat diet? http://www.nutritionandmetabolism.com/content/2/1/27.

Feinman RD, Fine EJ. "A calorie is a calorie" violates the second law of thermodynamics. http:// www.nutritionj.com/content/3/1/9.

Flynn M, Sciamanna C and Vigilante K. Inadequate physician knowledge of the effects of diet on blood lipids and lipoproteins. http://www.nutritionjcom/content/2/1/19.

Fontaine KR, Redden DT, Wang C et al. Years of life lost due to obesity. JAMA 2003; 289: 187–93.

Ford ES and Liu S. Glycemic index and serum high-density lipoprotein cholesterol concentration among US adults. Arch Intern Med 2001; 161: 572–6.

Foster GD, Wyatt HR, Hill JO et al. A randomized trial of a low-carbohydrate diet for obesity. N Engl J Med 2003; 348: 2082–90.

Freedland ES. Role of critical visceral adipose tissue threshold (CVATT) in metabolic syndrome: Implications for controlling dietary carbohydrates: A review. http://www.nutritionandmetabolism.com/content/1/1/12.

Freeman JM, Kossoff EH and Hartman AL. The ketogenic diet: One decade later. Pedriatrics 2007; 119: 535–43.

Galofré JC, Pujante P, Abreu C et al. Relationship between thyroidstimulating hormone and insulin in euthyroid obese men. Ann Nutr Metab 2008; 53: 188–94.

Gannon MC and Nuttol FQ. Effect of a high-protein, low-carbohydrate diet on blood glucose control in people with type 2 diabetes. Diabetes 2004; 53: 2375–82.

Gardner CD, Kiazand A, Alhassan S et al. Comparison of the Atkins, Zone, Ornish, and LEARN diets for change in weight and related risk factors among overweight premenopausal women. JAMA 2007; 297: 969–77.

German JB, Gibson RA, Krauss RM et al. A reprisal of the impact of dairy foods and milk fat on cardiovascular disease risk. Eur J Nutr 2009; 48: 191–203.

Glimcher LH and Lee AH. From sugar to fat: How the transcription factor XBP1 regulates hepatic lipogenesis. Ann N Y Acad Sci 2009; 1173 Suppl 1: E2–9.

Gross LS, Li L, Ford ES et al. Increased consumption of refined carbohydrates and the epidemic of type 2 diabetes in the United States: An ecologic assessment. Am J Clin Nutr 2004; 79: 774–9.

Grover SA, Lowensteyn I, Kaouache M et al. The prevalence of erectile dysfunction in the primary care setting. Arch Intern Med 2006; 166: 213–9.

Gunter MJ, Hoover DR, Yu H et al. Insulin, insulin-like growth factor-I, and risk of breast cancer in postmenopausal women. J Natl Cancer Inst 2009; 7: 48–60.

Halton TL, Willett WC, Liu S et al. Low-carbohydrate-diet score and the risk of coronary heart disease in women. N Engl J Med 2006; 355: 1991–2002.

He K, Merchant A, Rimm EB et al. Dietary fat intake and risk of stroke in male US healthcare professionals: 14 year prospective cohort study. BMJ 2003; 327: 777–82.

Heller S. Weight gain during insulin therapy in patients with type 2 diabetes mellitus. Diabet Res Clin Pract 2004; 65S: S23–7.

Henry RR and Gumbiner B. Benefits and limitations of very-low-calorie diet therapy in obese NDDM. Diabetes Care 1991; 14: 802–23.

Hertzler SR, Kim Y. Glycemic and insulenemic response to energy bars of differing macronutritient composition in healthy adults. Medical Science Monitor 2003; 9: CR84-90.

Hexeberg S. Ekstrem vektreduksjon uten kirurgi. Tidsskr Nor Legeforen 2009; 129: 2497.

Hexeberg S og Lindberg FA. Kvinnelig insulinbruker med diabetes type 2 og vektproblemer. Tidsskr Nor Legeforen 2008; 128: 443-5.

Holmberg S, Thelin A and Stiernström E-L et al. Food choices and coronary heart disease: A population based cohort study of rural swedish men with 12 years of follow-up. Int J Environ Res Public Health 2009; 6: 2626-38.

Hopkinson ZEC, Sattar N, Fleming R et al. Polycystic ovarian syndrome: The metabolic syndrome comes to gynaecology. BMJ 1998; 317: 329-32.

Howard BV, Van Horn L, Hsia J et al. Low-fat dietary pattern and risk of cardiovascular disease. The women's health initiative randomized controlled dietary modification trial. JAMA 2006; 295: 655-66.

Hsu LK, Crisp AH, Kalucy RS et al. Early morning migraine. Nocturnal plasma levels of catecholamines, tryptophan, glucose, and free fatty acids and sleep encephalographs. Lancet 1977; 26: 447-51.

Hudgins LC, Hellerstein M, Seidman C et al. Human fatty acid synthesis is stimulated by a eucaloric low fat, high carbohydrate diet. J Clin Invest 1996; 97: 2081-91.

Jee SH, Ohrr H, Sull JW et al. Fasting serum glucose level and cancer risk in korean men and women. JAMA 2005; 293: 194-202.

Kaaja R, Tikkanen MJ, Viinikka L et al. Serum lipoproteins, insulin, and urinary prostanoid metabolites in normal and hypertensive pregnant women. Obstet Gynecol 1995; 85: 353-6.

Kaya C, Yilmaz G, Nurkalem Z et al. Sexual function in women with coronary artery disease: A preliminary study. Int J Impot Res 2007; 19: 326–9.

Kahn SE, Zinman B, Haffner et al. Obesity is a major determinant of the association of C-reactive protein levels and the metabolic syndrom in type 2 diabetes. Diabetes 2006; 55: 2357–64.

Kandaraki E, Christakou C and Diamante-Kandarakis E. Metabolic syndrome and polycystic ovary syndrome... and vice versa. Arq Bras Endocrinol Metab 2009; 53: 227–37.

Kelwick A and Pawan GLS. Calorie intake in relation to body-weight changes in the obese. Lancet 1956; 268; 155–161.

Kelly CCJ, Lyall H, Petrie JR et al. Low grade chronic inflammation in women with polycystic ovarian syndrome. J Clin Endocrinol Metab 2001; 86: 2453–5.

Kirk JK, Graves DE, Craven TE et al. Restricted-carbohydrate diets in patients with type 2 diabetes: A meta-analysis. J Am Diet Assoc 2008; 108: 91–100.

Konradsen S, Ag H, Lindberg F et al. Serum 1,25-dihydroxy vitamin D is inversely associated with body mass index. Eur J Nutr 2008; 47: 87–91.

Kopp W. High-insulinogenic nutrition – an etiologic factor for obesity and the metabolic syndrome? Metabolism 2003; 52: 840–4.

Kritchevsky SB and Kritchevsky D. Egg consumption and coronary heart disease: An epidemiologic overview. J Am Coll Nutr 2000; 19: 549S–55S.

Kumar HK, Yadav RK, Prajapati J et al. Association between thyroid hormones, insulin resistance, and metabolic syndrome. Saudi Med J 2009; 30: 907–11.

Lakka H-M, Salonen JT, Tuomilehto J et al. Obesity and weight gain are associated with increased incidence of hyperinsulinemia in nondiabetic men. Horm Metab Res 2002; 34: 492–8.

Liu S, Manson JE, Stampfer MJ et al. Dietary glycemic load

assessed by food-frequency questionaire in relation to plasma high-density-lipoprotein cholesterol and fasting plasma triacylglycerols in postmenopausal women. Am J Clin Nutr 2001; 73: 560–6.

Liu S, Willett WC, Stampfer MJ et al. A prospective study of dietary glycemic load, carbohydrate intake, and risk of coronary heart disease in US women. Am J Clin Nutr 2000; 71: 1455–61.

Loevinger BL, Muller D, Aloso et al. Metabolic syndrome in women with chronic pain. Metabolism 2007; 56; 87–93.

Lyons TJ, Bailie KE, Dyer DG et al. Decrease in skin collagen glycation with improved glycemic control in patients with insulin-dependent diabetes mellitus. J Clin Invest 1991; 87: 1910–5.

Maedler K, Sergeev P, Ris F et al. Glucose-induced β cell production of IL-1ß contributes to glucotoxicity in human pancreatic islets. J Clin Invest 2002; 110; 851–60.

Margioris AN. Fatty acids and postprandial inflammation. Curr Opin Clin Nutr Metab Care 2009; 12: 129–37.

Marfella R, Esposito K, Giunta R et al. Circulating adhesion molecules in humans: Role of hyperglycemia and hyperinsulinemia. Circulation 2000; 101: 2247–51.

Marfella R, Quagliaro L, Nappo F et al. Acute hyperglycemia induces an oxidative stress in healthy subjects. J Clin Invest 2001; 108: 635–6.

Marks R and Allegrante JP. Body mass indices in patients with disabling hip osteoarthtritis. Arthritis Res 2002; 4: 112–6.

Martin WF, Armstrong LE and Rodriguez NR. Dietary protein intake and renal function.
http://www.nutritionandmetabolism.com/content/2/1/25.

Mavropoulos JC, Yancy WS, Hepburn J et al. The effects of a low-carbohydrate, ketogenic diet on the polycystic ovary syndrome: A pilot study.
http://www.nutritionandmetabolism.com/content/2/1/35.

Meigs JB, Nathan DM, D'Agostino RB et al. Fasting and postchallenge glycemia and cardiovascular disease risk. Diabetes Care 2002; 25: 1845–50.

Michalaki MA, Vagenakis AG, Leonardou AS et al. Thyroid function in humans with morbid obesity. Thyroid 2006; 16: 73–8.

Misciagana G, Guerra V, Di Leo A et al. Insulin and gall stones: A population case control study in southern Italy. Gut 2000; 47: 144–7.

Moan J og Porojnicu AC. D-vitaminets fotobiologi – ny aktualitet. Tidsskr Nor Legeforen 2006; 8: 1048–52.

Mozaffarian D, Rimm EB, Herrington DM. Dietary fats, carbohydrate, and progression of coronary atherosclerosis in postmenopausal women. Am J Clin Nutr 2004; 80: 1175–1184.

Mueller A, Schöfl C, Dittrich R et al. Thyroid-stimulating hormone is associated with insulin resistance independently of body mass index and age in women with polycystic ovary syndrome. Hum Reprod 2009; 24: 2924–39.

Muniyappa R, Montagnani M, Kon Koh K et al. Cardiovascular actions of insulin. Endocr Rev 2007; 28: 463–91.

Newkirk MM, Goldbach-Mansky R, Lee J et al. Advanced glycation end-product (AGE)-damaged IgG and IgM autoantibodies to IgG-AGE in patients with early synovitis. Arthritis Res Ter 2003; 5: R82–90.

Nielsen FH, Milne DB, Klevay LM et al. Dietary magnesium deficiency induces heart rhytm changes, impairs glucose tolerance, and decreases serum cholesterol in post menopausal women. J American Coll Nutr 2007; 26: 121–32.

Nielsen JV and Joensson E. Low-carbohydrate diet in type 2 diabetes. Stable improvement of bodyweight and glycemic control during 22 months follow-up. http://www.nutritionandmetabolism.com/content/3/1/22.

Nielsen JV and Joensson EA. Low-carbohydrate diet in type 2

diabetes: Stable improvement of bodyweight and glycemic control during 44 months follow-up. http://www.nutritionandmetabolism.com/content/5/1/14.

Odeley OE, de Courton M, Pettitt DJ et al. Fasting hyperinsulinemia is a predictor of increased body weight gain and obesity in prima indian children. Diabetes 1997; 46: 1341–5.

Oh SY, Kang MS, Yoo TW et al. The association between increased alanine aminotransferase activity and metabolic factors in nonalcoholic fatty liver disease. Metabolism 2006; 55: 1604–9.

Pereira MA, Swain J, Goldfine AB et al. Effects of a low-glycemic load diet on resting energy expenditure and heart disease risk factors during weight loss. JAMA 2004; 292: 2482–90.

Peterline BL, Bigal ME, Tepper SJ et al. Migraine and adiponectin: Is there a connection? Cephalagia 2007: 27: 435–46.

Phinney SD. Ketogenic diets and physical performance. http://www.nutritionandmetabolism.com/content/1/1/2.

Pittas AG, Dawson-Hughes B, Li T et al. Vitamin D and calcium intake in relation to type 2 diabetes in women. Diabetes Care 2006; 29: 650–6.

Poleszynski DV, Mysterud I, Lindberg FA m.fl. Myndighetenes ernæringsråd bør revideres. Tidsskr Nor Legeforen 2009; 129: 2382–4.

Rainero I, Limone P, Ferrero M et al. Insulin sensitivity is impaired in patients with migraine. Cephalagia 2005; 25: 593–7.

Ratliff JC, Mutungi G, Puglisi MJ et al. Eggs modulate the inflammatory response to carbohydrate restricted diets in overweight men. http://www.nutritionandmetabolism.com/content/5/1/6.

Robker RL, Akison LK, Bennett BD et al. Obese women exhibit differences in ovarian metabolites, hormones, and gene expression compared with moderate-weight women. J Clin Endocrinol Metab 2009; 94: 1533–40.

Roos A, Bakker SJL, Links TP et al. Thyroid function is associated with components of the metabolic syndrom in euthyroid subjects. J Clin Endocrinol Metab 2007; 92: 491–6.

Rotondi M, Leporati P, La Manna A et al. Raised serum TSH levels in patients with morbid obesity: Is it enough to diagnose subclinical hypothyroidisme? Eur J Endocrinol 2009; 160: 403–8.

Rubinstein I, Slutsky AS, Zamel N et al. Paradoxical glottis narrowing in patients with severe obstructive sleep apnea. J Clin Invest 1988; 81: 1051–5.

Ruderman N, Chisholm D, Pi-Sunyer X et al. The metabolically obese, normal-weight individual revisited. Diabetes 1998; 47: 699–713.

Sam S, Haffner S, Davidson MH et al. Relationship of abdominal visceral and subcutaneous adipose tissue with lipoprotein particle number and size in type 2 diabetes. Diabetes 2008; 57: 222–7.

Samaha FF, Iqbal N, Seshadri P et al. A low-carbohydrate as compared with a low-fat diet in severe obesity. N Engl J Med 2003; 348: 2074–81.

Sampson MJ, Davies IR, Brown JC et al. Monocyte and neutrophil adhesion molecule expression during acute hyperglycemia and after antioxidant treatment in type 2 diabetes and control patients. Arterioscler Thromb Vasc Biol 2002; 22: 1187–93.

Sauvaget C, Nagano J, Hayashi M et al. Animal protein, animal fat, and cholesterol intakes and risk of cerebral infarction mortality in the adult health study. Stroke 2004; 35: 1531–7.

Savage DB, Petersen KF and Shulman GI. Mechanisms of insulin resistance in humans and possible links with inflammation. Hypertension 2005; 45: 828–33.

Schenk S, Saberi M and Olefsky JM et al. Insulin sensitivity:

Modulation by nutritions and inflammation. J Clin invest 2008; 118: 2992–3002.

Scherrer U, Randin D, Vollenweider P et al. Nitric oxide release accounts for insulin's vascular effects in humans. J Clin Invest 1994; 94: 2511–5.

Schwartz J-M, Linfoot P, Dare D et al. Hepatic de novo lipogenesis in normoinsulinemic and hyperinsulinemic subjects consuming highfat, low-carbohydrate and low-fat, high carbohydrate isoenergetic diets. Am J Clin Nutr 2003; 77: 43–50.

Scoll TO and Chen X. Insulin and the "thrifty" woman: The influence of insulin during pregnancy on gestational weight gain and postpartum weight retention. Matern Child Health J 2002; 6: 255–61.

Shaw JE, Hodge AM, de Courten M et al. Isolated post-challenge hyperglycaemia confirmed as a risk factor for mortality. Diabetologia 199; 42: 1050–4.

Seely EW and Solomon CG. Insulin resisteance and its potential role in pregnancy-induced hypertension. J Clin Endocrinol 2003; 88: 2393–8.

Selvin E, Coresh J, Golden SH et al. Glycemic control and coronary heart disease risk in persons with and without diabetes. Arch Intern Med 2005; 165: 1910–6.

Seshadri P, Iqbal N, Stern L et al. A randomized study comparing the effects of a low-carbohydrate diet and a conventional diet on lipoprotein subfractions and C-reactive protein levels in patients with severe obesity. Am J med 2004; 15: 398–405.

Shai I, Schwarzfuchs D, Henkin Y et al. Weight loss with low-carbohydrate, mediterranean, or low-fat diet. N Eng J Med 2008; 359: 229–41.

Shanta GPS, Kumar AA, Jeyachandran et al. Association between primary hypothyroidism and metabolic syndrome and the role of C reactive protein: A cross-sectional study

from South India.
http://www.thyroidresearchjournal.com/content/2/1/2.

Sharman MJ, Kraemer WJ, Love DM et al. A ketogenic diet favorable affects serum biomarkers for cardiovascular disease in normal-weight men. J Nutr 2002; 132: 1879–85.

Ship J. Diabetes and oral health. JADA 2003; 134: 4S–10S.

Sigal RJ, El-Hashimy M, Martin BC et al. Acute postchallenge hyperinsulinemi predicts weight gain. Diabetes 1997; 46: 1025–9.

Siri PW, Krauss RM. Influence of dietary carbohydrate and fat on LDL and HDL particle distributions. Curr. Atheroscler Rep 2005; 7: 455–9.

Siri-Tarino PW, Qi S, Hu FB et al. Meta-analysis of prospective cohort studies evaluating the association of saturated fat with cardiovascular disease. Am J Clin Nutr 2010; doc: 10–3945/ajcn. 2009. 27725.

Smedman AEM, Gustafsson I-G, Berglund LGT et al. Pentadecanoic acid in serum as a marker for intake of milk fat: Relations between intake of milk fat and metabolic risk factors. Am J Clin Nutr 1999; 69: 22–9.

Stattin P, Björ O, Ferrari P et al. Prospective study of hyperglycemia and cancer risk. Diabetes Care 2007; 30: 561–7.

Stratton IM, Adler AI, Neil HAW et al. Association of glycaemia with macrovascular and microvascular complications of type 2 diabetes (UKPDS 35): prospective observational study. BMJ 2000; 321: 405–412.

Tishler M, Smorodin T, Vazina-Amit M et al. Fibromyalgia in diabetes mellitus. Rhematol Int 2003; 23: 171–3.

Trauninger A, Pfund Z, Koszegi T et al. Oral magnesium load test in patients with migraine. Headache 2002; 42: 114–9.

Tsai C-J, Leitzmann MF, Willett WC et al. Dietary carbohydrates and glycaemic load and the incidence of symptomatic gall stone disease in men. Gut 2005; 54: 823–8.

Turina M, Fry DE and Polk HC. Acute hyperglycemia and the innate immune system: Clinical, cellular, and molecular aspects. Crit Care Med 2005; 33: 1624–33.

Vanhala M, Vanhala P, Kumpusola E et al. Relation between obesity from childhood to adulthood and the metabolic syndrome: Population based study. BMJ 1998; 317: 9.

Van Oss CJ. Influence of glucose levels on the in vitro phagocytosis of bacteria by human neutrophils. Infect Immun 1971; 4: 54–9.

Visser J, Rozing J, Sapone A et al. Tight Junctions, intestinal permeability, and autoimmunity. Ann NY Acad Sci 2009; 1165: 195–205.

Volek JS, Sharman MJ, Gómez AL et al. Comparison of energy-restricted very low-carbohydrate and low-fat diets on weight loss and body composition in overweight men and women. http://www.nutritionandmetabolism.com/content/1/1/13.

Volek JS, Sharman MJ, Gómez AL et al. An isoenergetic very low carbohydrate diet improves serum HDL cholesterol and triacylglycerol concentrations, the total cholesterol to HDL cholesterol ratio and postprandial lipemic responses compared with a low fat diet in normal weight, normolipidemic women. J Nutr 2003; 133: 2756–61.

Volek JS and Feinman RD. Carbohydrate restriction improves the features of metabolic syndrome. Metabolic syndrome may be defined by the response to carbohydrate restriction. http://www.nutritionandmetabolism.com/content/2/1/31.

Volek JS, Gómez AL and Kraemer WJ. Fasting lipoprotein and postprandial triacylglycerol responses to a low-carbohydrate diet supplemented with n-3 fatty acids. J Am Coll Nutr 2000; 19: 383–91.

Westman EC, Yancy Jr WS, Mavropoulos JC et al. The effect of a lowcarbohydrate, ketogenic diet versus a low-glycemic index diet on glycemic control in type 2 diabetes mellitus. http://www.nutritionandmetabolism.com/content/5/1/36.

Weyer C, Hanson RL, Tataranni A et al. A high fasting plasma insulin concentration predicts type 2 diabetes independent of insulin resistance. Diabetes 2000; 49: 2094–2100.

Wolk R, Shamsuzzaman ASM, Somers VK. Obesity, sleep apnea, and hypertension. Hypertension 2003; 42: 1067–74.

Yancy Jr WS, Marjorie F, Chalecki AM et al. A low-carbohydrate, ketogenic diet to treat type 2 diabetes. http://www.nutritionandmetabolism.com/content/2/1/34.

Yost TJ, Jensen DR, Haugen BR et al. Effect of dietary macronutrient composition on tissue-spesific lipoprotein lipase activity and insulin action in normal-weight subjects. Am J Clin Nutr 1998; 68: 296–302.

Yudkin JS, Stehouwer CDA, Emeis JJ et al. C-reaktive protein in healthy subjects: Association with obesity, insulin resistance, and endothelial dysfunction: A potential role for cytokines originating from adipose tissue? Arterioscler Thromb Vasc Biol 1999; 19: 972–8.

Please visit

http://www.thescandinaviandiet.com/